Health Disparities

Adam Perzynski • Sarah Shick
Ifeolorunbode Adebambo

Editors

Health Disparities

Weaving a New Understanding Through
Case Narratives

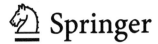

Editors
Adam Perzynski
Case Western Reserve University
Center for Health Care Research
and Policy, The MetroHealth System
Cleveland, OH, USA

Sarah Shick
Department of Sociology
Case Western Reserve University
Center for Health Care Research
and Policy, The MetroHealth System
Cleveland, OH, USA

Ifeolorunbode Adebambo
Case Western Reserve University
Cleveland, OH, USA

ISBN 978-3-030-12773-2   ISBN 978-3-030-12771-8   (eBook)
https://doi.org/10.1007/978-3-030-12771-8

This Springer imprint is published by the registered company Springer Nature Switzerland AG
The registered company address is: Gewerbestrasse 11, 6330 Cham, Switzerland

This book is dedicated to our patients and their families. Their stories of pain and struggle scream out for equity in health.

My Endorsement for Health Disparities and Social Determinants: Weaving a New Understanding Through Case Narratives

I was impressed when I read *Health Disparities and Social Determinants: Weaving a New Understanding Through Case Narratives.* As a patient who has experienced unpleasant situations in health care, I was moved to see that it was emotional and personal for the writers. The book confirms for me that the time is now for change to take place in our health-care systems. I see this book as a light that can shine bright in the darkest places of health care. The editors have assembled a powerful book that provides all professionals in the health-care systems with specific steps they can take toward addressing and then eventually eliminating health disparities. A few steps that I really connected with were improve critical awareness, deliver quality of care, listen and empathize with patients and families, and advocate for changes. I recommend obtaining a copy of this book to everyone interested in working to improve health care because it's filled with useful information that every medical professional should know. The book reminds me of a quote by Wayne Dyer, "When you change the way you look at things, the things you look at change."

– Delores Collins aka Ms. Dee, Founder and Executive Director, A Vision of Change Incorporated, Certified Community Health Worker, Founder of The Greater Cleveland Community Health Workers Association

November 21, 2018

Preface

This book is a challenge. It is a challenge to you and to me and to our brothers and sisters and neighbors. The book begs us to figure out how we can do better in health care. On May 24, 2018, I sat in my backyard editing some of the contributions from generous individuals who took the time to write down their thoughts, experiences, and tragedies and failures. Once again, I cried. Most often, it is after reading a specific narrative that my tear ducts open and grief floods my mind. On this day though, it was the sheer magnitude of everything in this book together. Sometimes the book has made me angry; sometimes it is a story, and sometimes, of all things, I am angry at the person who wrote one of the stories. How could they say that! Some of these narratives are raw in their content and form. So much so that you might think critically of the author or of the editors. Good. This book sprouted from a seed in a garden of narrative humility. Your critical thoughts and reactions are an asset we hope to unearth as you pass through the stories.

The very first time Dr. Adebambo (Bode) and I gave a health disparity workshop, we were with a group of about 30 Internal Medicine residents. They read the narrative titled, "Time to Leave." During that workshop and dozens of seminars, learning sessions, and workshops since, we have seen a pallor of quiet reflection befall the room. We have heard anger and frustration.

In that first session, a resident volunteered his opinion of one of the patients, "I think all of this was just her fault."

Immediately, one of his peers countered, "How could you possibly say that?! You do not even understand what she has had to go through in her life and you have the nerve to say that it was all her fault?"

The tension, challenge, and discomfort that happen in our workshops will surely happen to readers of this book and in courses, seminars, and classrooms where students find themselves reading these narratives. Good. The social and emotional learning that can be discovered in stories like "Time to Leave" is almost impossible to acquire from a solely quantitative, fact-based approach. Teachers, faculty, and workshop facilitators will likely want to spend some time reviewing the last several chapters of the book before assigning narratives to their students. Students might also benefit from reviewing the last several chapters in order to grasp for themselves the pedagogical techniques that are being implemented in their own education.

Assembling this book over so many years, I have occasionally reflected on Ovid's account of the story of Philomela. According to the myth, Philomela was forcibly taken to a cabin in the woods and raped by Tereus. Philomela was defiant and refused to keep quiet about the rape. Tereus cut out her tongue. Unable to speak, Philomela wove a tapestry to tell her story. This part of the tale of Philomela is oft referred to as "The Voice of the Shuttle" (the shuttle being the tool that is moved back and forth through the loom during weaving). This book is not so much a telling but a weaving together of the daily, silent tragedies that are happening in health care today.

A colleague of mine, April Urban, once remarked on Twitter, "Sometimes the problems are just too big." I interpret this as less of a statement about the problems themselves and more of a statement about the daunting challenge of solving very serious, very complex, and very urgent problems. This book is here now because we need to talk more about the problems. We need to talk about how health disparities happen and how we can work together to find solutions to health disparities and pathways to address social needs. Sarah, Bode, and I offer this book to you, in all humility, as a starting point for learning, action, and reflection.

Acknowledgments

For their leadership and support of this effort, we would like to thank Dr. Aleece Caron, Dr. James Campbell, Dr. Ashwini Sehgal, Dr. John Boltri, Dr. Joseph Sudano, Dr. Francine Hekelman, and Maria Zebrowski. We further extend our thanks to all of the patients, families, and community members who have inspired our work and contributed to review of this volume. We also thank Megan Hammond, MEd for her help and support with the depiction of what women with spinal cord injury face when accessing health care.

This book was made possible through the accomplishments of the scholars and faculty participating in the "Primary Care Faculty Development Program" (HRSA: D55HP23193, James Campbell, MD, Principal Investigator) and two spinoff projects, "Primary Care Training Enhancement" for faculty and residents (HRSA 1 T0BHP285570100, Aleece Caron PhD, Principal Investigator) and "Advancing Primary Care Competency Across the Training Continuum in Northeast Ohio's Rural and Underserved Communities" (HRSA 1 T0BHP30006010 John Boltri, MD, Principal Investigator). Further support was provided by the NINR-funded study, "Targeted Management Intervention for African-American Men with TIA or Stroke" (TEAM Study; 1R21NR013001, Martha Sajatovic, Principal Investigator).

Cleveland, OH, USA   Adam Perzynski

Contents

Introduction

Adam Perzynski and Francine Hekelman

This book seeks to provide an initial framework for promoting learning about health disparities and social determinants of health among health professionals. In 2012, we began to teach health disparities to primary care physicians as part of a faculty development program. During the delivery of the health disparities component of the program, we developed a range of teaching strategies, curricula, and associated resources for promoting learning about health disparities among medical professionals. In this chapter we provide an overview of possible goals and objectives for a health disparities curriculum and an introduction to our pedagogical approach.

Background

MetroHealth Medical Center is an urban, county-funded, safety net public hospital and a Level I trauma center in Cleveland, Ohio. Since its beginning in 1837, MetroHealth's constituents have disproportionately represented the poor, the elderly, people of many different races and ethnicities, and others from the City of Cleveland and Cuyahoga County who are in need of health care and often unable to pay. In addition, MetroHealth is known for a wide range of medical programs that treat patients with burns, kidney failure, tuberculosis, and HIV/AIDS and infants of addicted mothers, a physical medicine and rehabilitation department notable for care of spinal cord injury and traumatic brain injury and a bustling

A. Perzynski
Center for Health Care Research and Policy, The MetroHealth System, Case Western Reserve University, Cleveland, OH, USA

F. Hekelman (✉)
The MetroHealth System, Cleveland, OH, USA
e-mail: fhekelman@metrohealth.org

© The Author(s) 2019
A. Perzynski et al. (eds.), *Health Disparities*,
https://doi.org/10.1007/978-3-030-12771-8_1

emergency room. MetroHealth is an affiliated Institution of Case Western Reserve University (CWRU). Narratives in this book draw upon decades of experience from clinicians caring for patients at MetroHealth and at many clinics, hospitals, and community locations in Cleveland and across Ohio and other areas.

The Department of Family Medicine at MetroHealth was the academic hub for educating three to four faculty scholars per year in an effort to develop basic knowledge, skills, and attitudes essential to medical scholarship. To this day, the overall curriculum of our training and faculty development programs consists of four primary courses including medical education, health disparities and social determinants, population health, and quality improvement. While this book relies primarily on narratives and innovations in health disparities education, we also experienced a synthesis from other collaborating educators in developing objectives, content, instructional methods, evaluation methods, and other features of the health disparities curriculum. Our work benefits most especially from the insights, writing, and ideas that come from faculty scholar learners themselves.

Goals of the Health Disparities Curriculum

The overall goals of the health disparities curriculum are similar to those typically found in undergraduate and graduate university coursework, and those are echoed here in this book. We review clinical cases together with social, political, economic, cultural, legal, and ethical theories related to health disparities in order to:

1. Develop a nuanced understanding of causes of health disparities.
2. Describe how health-care system and individual issues coalesce to create health disparities.
3. Connect health disparities encountered in clinical medicine to broader social problems.
4. Explore strategies for reducing/eliminating health disparities.
5. Encourage scholars to learn self-directed positive habits of the mind in writing a case narrative on a specific patient with a health disparity or a specific social situation, thereby challenging the scholar to develop knowledge proficiency.

Preparation of a Health Disparities Curriculum

Preparation of materials for a health disparities curriculum presents a unique set of challenges. Existing graduate-level courses on health disparities, including one co-taught by Dr. Perzynski at CWRU, are targeted to an audience of graduate student learners who more often than not have little firsthand knowledge of health disparities. The situation is drastically different at MetroHealth where clinical personnel are confronted on a daily basis with adverse circumstances, including patients who live in poverty, are homeless, do not have health insurance or a regular source of income, and who come from a wide variety of diverse racial and ethnic backgrounds, many of whom do not speak English.

When planning our program in 2011, a search of the literature on teaching health disparities and social determinants of health to current and future health-care practitioners yielded few results. In the absence of a strong literature supporting educational strategies for health disparities in this audience, our approach was to rework the aforementioned graduate-level health disparities course by enlisting the input of the learners, the clinical faculty in the faculty development program.

Emergent Learning

Our emergent learning approach is adapted from the book, *We Are All Explorers,* which describes the *Reggio Amelia* approach to education that has been successful among young school children (Scheinfeld et al. 2008). According to the *Reggio Amelia* approach, people learn best when they explore a topic out of their own desire to know more about it. Thus, among our learners the curriculum is structured to elicit the scholars' own experiences and concerns about health disparities first and then select readings and craft a set of activities "on the fly." For example, in the introductory health disparities session it became clear that the seminar participants had a great deal to say about their direct experiences and frustrations with how broader social problems can become health disparities for their patients.

In response to this interest, participants were asked to draft case narratives of the social needs and disparities encountered by patients in their clinical practice. We designed a miniature curriculum that taught the scholars the principles of developing and writing case narratives with a focus on health disparities and social needs. The problem of not knowing the best ways to teach doctors about health disparities became the responsibility of the learners, and the process of learning about health disparities also became a process of collaborative learning of how to teach others.

In addition, the learners have gone on to develop and implement workshops and curricula for (1) teaching health disparities through narrative among Advanced Practice Registered Nurses via simple workshops; (2) promoting learning about health disparities among physician residents and trainees in a mini-course structure as part of residency; (3) developing curricula and materials for workshops at national health professional meetings, including one given at the 2014 Annual Meeting of the Society for Teachers of Family Medicine and another at The American Geriatrics Society Annual Meeting; (4) developing their own new health disparities courses in medical schools and clinical departments around the country; and (5) implementing dozens of new quality improvement and research projects focused on addressing social determinants of health in care processes and disease outcomes.

The case narrative approach provides opportunity for ongoing reflective critique and revisions. While the emergent learning approach has many advantages, on occasion the participants and the instructors struggled slightly with the loose, exploratory learning environment. For example, faculty scholars' feedback indicated that they craved more structure in the curriculum, including a preference for more detailed and structured handouts. Thus, changes were made to supplement the open, seminar atmosphere with more detailed handouts and some other more structured activities including the viewing of videos on health disparities and visits by local health disparities experts.

The demands of health and medical training and the pace of work in clinical environments caused some participants to have difficulties fitting writing into their schedules. As instructors, we have found it challenging to provide timely feedback on the written cases prepared by participants. We worked to spend additional in-class time devoted to writing, and class time was occasionally "traded" to the scholars in order that they were able to spend additional time writing and revising their written case narratives. In all, the challenges of the emergent learning approach are more than outweighed by the benefits to the scholars' learning and changes in attitudes about health disparities. The broad enthusiasm among the scholars for sharing our work on health disparities with local and national audiences has been particularly encouraging.

Objectives from Health Disparities and Social Determinants Narrative Workshops

In exchange for the opportunity to participate in learning activities, participants are expected to:

1. Define and understand the nature of health disparities and social determinants of health as they affect patients and families of lower economic situations, patients of diverse racial and ethnic groups, and other disadvantaged populations.
2. Learn how to prepare a case narrative of a specific patient based upon oral and written feedback from faculty and fellow scholars.
3. Submit the case narrative for review and comment by the session leader.
4. Present the case narrative to the class for discussion, clarification, and feedback.
5. Revise the narrative and place it in his/her electronic portfolio.
6. Evaluate what s/he learned from the case narrative and the presentation to the class.
7. Commit to include the case narrative in future publications or presentations.

Evaluation and Outcomes for the Faculty Case Narratives Component

Over the last 6 years, hundreds of learners in our programs and courses have read, written, and/or presented a case narrative. Based on this writing, many have gone on to submit abstracts, give oral presentations, conduct workshops, redesign residency curricula, conduct quality improvement or research projects, and even develop new clinical and academic programs.

Each time such an occasion has occurred, scholars have discussed the presentation as well as the results shared by each of the participants through their evaluations and feedback. As we continued to develop the program, we realized that many of these narratives were useful teaching tools and could be adapted for other health professionals, especially if we developed a collection that included an array of tools and learning experiences. Our overall goal is to eliminate health disparities. The pathway to that goal includes a critical awareness of the problem, a desire to improve the quality of care delivered to individuals of disadvantaged backgrounds, and the skills and resources to help team members understand their role in listening and empathizing with patients and families, as well as documenting and advocating for changes in social determinants of health.

At the outset, we did not realize that our work would become a model for teaching diverse learners in a variety of settings. True to form in the *Reggio* method, we are *all* explorers, and the process of learning about social determinants and discovering how to best promote awareness of health disparities continues through a shared sense of responsibility to sponsor health and social equity. We hope that the gentle minds of everyone who reads this book, from learners to workshop facilitators and faculty, experience growth in learning and passion that spreads throughout medical schools, health professions programs, and health institutions. We as professionals have a need to understand the social and cultural implications of disparities and determine a plan of action to effectively address social determinants and eliminate disparities in care and outcomes.

Reference

Scheinfeld DR, Haigh KM, Scheinfeld SJ (2008) We are all explorers: learning and teaching with Reggio principles in urban settings. Teachers College Press, New York

Health Disparities and Social Determinants of Health

Sarah Shick, Ifeolorunbode Adebambo, and Adam Perzynski

> *It is not our differences that divide us. It is our inability to recognize, accept, and celebrate those differences.*
>
> *There is no such thing as a single-issue struggle because we do not live single-issue lives.*
> *–Audre Lorde*

The narratives in this section are written by fellow physicians, nurses, and social scientists to demonstrate how health disparities influence care and create challenges for providers and patients alike. As the above Audre Lorde quotes suggests, recognizing and accepting the diverse, layered experiences of patients can lead to better care and a better experience for all involved.

In a story similar to one of the patients featured in the following narratives, Audre Lorde gained fame for her writings exploring on her experience as an African American lesbian with cancer and how it affected both her medical care and her interaction with the world. A thorough understanding of health disparities and the social determinants of health begins with some basic definitions.

Healthy People 2020 defines a health disparity as:

a particular type of health difference that is closely linked with social, economic, and/or environmental disadvantage. Health disparities adversely affect groups of people who have systematically experienced greater obstacles to health based on their racial or ethnic group; religion; socioeconomic status; gender; age; mental health; cognitive, sensory, or

S. Shick (✉)
Department of Sociology, Case Western Reserve University, Center for Health Care Research and Policy, The MetroHealth System, Cleveland, OH, USA
e-mail: ses165@case.edu

I. Adebambo
Department of Family Medicine, The MetroHealth System, Cleveland, OH, USA

A. Perzynski
Center for Health Care Research and Policy, The MetroHealth System, Case Western Reserve University, Cleveland, OH, USA

© The Author(s) 2019
A. Perzynski et al. (eds.), *Health Disparities*,
https://doi.org/10.1007/978-3-030-12771-8_2

physical disability; sexual orientation or gender identity; geographic location; or other characteristics historically linked to discrimination or exclusion. (Healthy People 2020 2018a)

The Kaiser Family Foundation further clarifies the difference between a health disparity and health-care disparity:

Health disparity: A higher burden of illness, injury, disability, or mortality experienced by one population group relative to another group.

Health care disparity: Differences between groups in health insurance coverage, access to and use of care, and quality of care. (Orgera and Artiga 2018)

The American Association of Family Practice (AAFP) has provided an important toolkit on the social determinants of health via the Everyone Project (Crawford 2018). The AAFP provides a simple and clear definition of social determinants:

The conditions under which people are born, grow, live, work, and age. (AAFP 2018)

Healthy People 2020 offers a similar definition:

Social determinants of health are conditions in the environments in which people are born, live, learn, work, play, worship, and age that affect a wide range of health, functioning, and quality-of-life outcomes and risks. (Healthy People 2020 2018b)

Social determinants can be further organized into five areas: economic stability, education, social and community context, health and health care, and the neighborhood or built environment (Healthy People 2020 2018b).

Example Data on Health Disparities

Health disparities are common and vary widely from place to place and across time periods. It is important to remember that disparities do not affect only racial and ethnic minorities but can impact any population depending on the health condition and other factors at play.

Healthy People 2020 provides an excellent online data resource for anyone interested in examining health disparities data across a wide array of social and demographic characteristics combined with disease and health-care process metrics. The *DATA 2020* tool (https://www.healthypeople.gov/2020/data-search/health-disparities-data) allows users to select a particular group characteristic (e.g. disability) and a particular outcome or process (e.g. health communication). In Figs. 1, 2, 3, 4, 5, 6, 7, 8, 9, 10, 11, 12, and 13, we present several examples of health disparities data across time and by subgroups. The web-based tool also allows users to narrow their data to individual states. Data are drawn from national health survey and surveillance resources like the National Health Interview Survey and the Medical Expenditure Panel Survey.

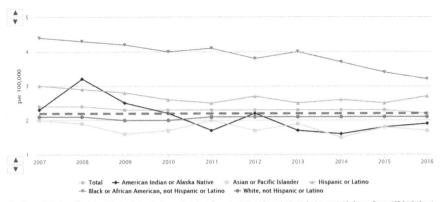

Data Source: Bridged-race Population Estimates; Centers for Disease Control and Prevention, National Center for Health Statistics and U.S. Census Bureau (CDC/NCHS and Census)

Fig. 1 Age-adjusted cervical cancer deaths per 100,000 population by race/ethnicity, 2007–2016. (Adapted from Healthy People 2020)

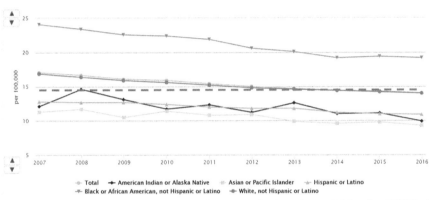

Data Source: Bridged-race Population Estimates; Centers for Disease Control and Prevention, National Center for Health Statistics and U.S. Census Bureau (CDC/NCHS and Census)

Fig. 2 Age-adjusted colon cancer deaths per 100,000 population by race/ethnicity, 2007–2016. (Adapted from Healthy People 2020)

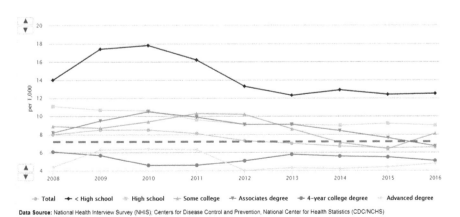

Data Source: National Health Interview Survey (NHIS); Centers for Disease Control and Prevention, National Center for Health Statistics (CDC/NCHS)

Fig. 3 New cases of diabetes among adults per 100,000 population by education level, 2008–2016. (Adapted from Healthy People 2020)

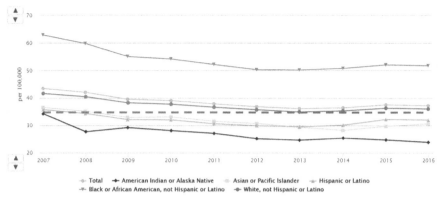

Data Source: Bridged-race Population Estimates; Centers for Disease Control and Prevention, National Center for Health Statistics and U.S. Census Bureau (CDC/NCHS and Census)
National Vital Statistics System-Mortality (NVSS-M); Centers for Disease Control and Prevention, National Center for Health Statistics (CDC/NCHS)

Fig. 4 Stroke deaths (age adjusted) per 100,000 population by race/ethnicity, 2007–2016. (Adapted from Healthy People 2020)

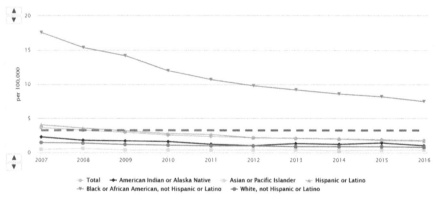

Data Source: National Vital Statistics System-Mortality (NVSS-M). Centers for Disease Control and Prevention, National Center for Health Statistics (CDC/NCHS)

Fig. 5 Deaths from HIV infection per 100,000 population by race/ethnicity, 2007–2016. (Adapted from Healthy People 2020)

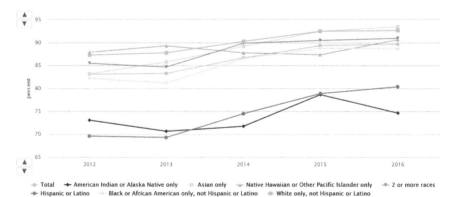

Data Source: National Health Interview Survey (NHIS); Centers for Disease Control and Prevention, National Center for Health Statistics (CDC/NCHS)

Fig. 6 Percent of persons under age 65 with medical insurance by race/ethnicity, 2012–2016. (Adapted from Healthy People 2020)

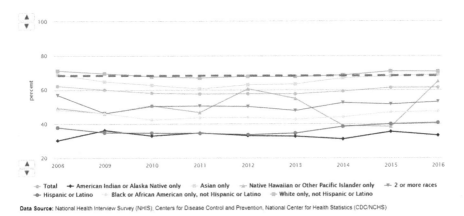

Data Source: National Health Interview Survey (NHIS), Centers for Disease Control and Prevention, National Center for Health Statistics (CDC/NCHS)

Fig. 7 Percent of persons under age 65 with prescription drug insurance by race/ethnicity, 2008–2016. (Adapted from Healthy People 2020)

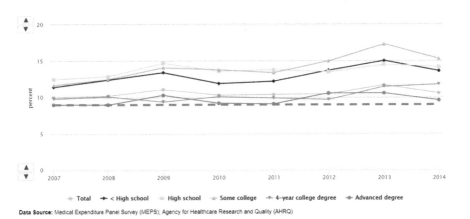

Data Source: Medical Expenditure Panel Survey (MEPS); Agency for Healthcare Research and Quality (AHRQ)

Fig. 8 Percent of persons unable to obtain needed medical care, dental care, or medications by educational attainment, 2007–2014. (Adapted from Healthy People 2020)

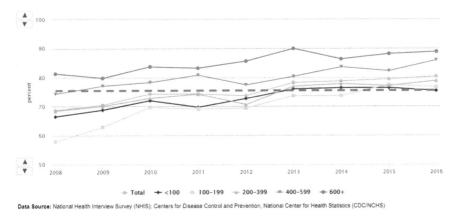

Data Source: National Health Interview Survey (NHIS); Centers for Disease Control and Prevention, National Center for Health Statistics (CDC/NCHS)

Fig. 9 Percent of adolescents (10–17 years) with a wellness checkup in the past 12 months by family income (percent poverty level), 2008–2016. (Adapted from Healthy People 2020)

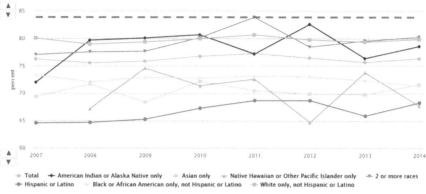

Fig. 10 Percent of persons with a usual primary care provider by race/ethnicity, 2007–2014. (Adapted from Healthy People 2020)

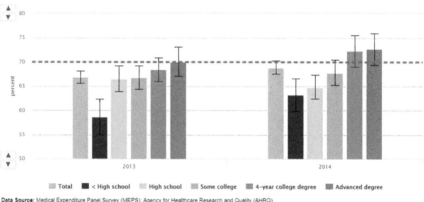

Fig. 11 Percent of persons whose healthcare provider gives easy-to-understand instructions by educational attainment, 2013–2014. (Adapted from Healthy People 2020)

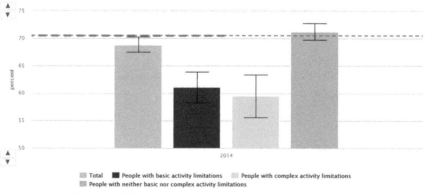

Fig. 12 Percent of persons whose healthcare provider gives easy-to-understand instructions by disability status, 2014. (Adapted from Healthy People 2020)

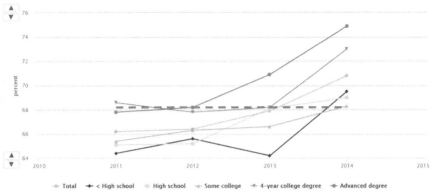

Fig. 13 Percent of persons whose healthcare provider always showed respect for what they have to say by educational attainment, 2011–2014. (Adapted from Healthy People 2020)

Example population trends in health disparities for cervical cancer, colon cancer, diabetes, stroke, and HIV are displayed in Figs. 1, 2, 3, 4, and 5. These nationwide data demonstrate a consistent overall decrease in the burden of disease over the last decade. Racial and ethnic (Figs. 1, 2, 4, and 5) and educational disparities (Fig. 3) are persistent but showing some small improvement. Although not shown in the example figures, it is important to note that outcome disparities can vary widely by sex and gender as well as by other characteristics. The concept of intersectionality is further useful for understanding such differences.

Despite the fact that health-care delivery and health disparities are experienced at the local level, many of the case narratives in the following chapters have clear linkages to the national disparities data presented in the figures. For example, the first narrative in this volume, "Time to Leave" describes a woman's experience with cervical cancer (Fig. 1).

In addition to health outcomes, there are clear and persistent disparities in health-care coverage (Fig. 6) and prescription drug coverage (Fig. 7). These gaps in coverage combined with rising health-care costs are no doubt related to the ongoing observed disparities in the decision to delay seeking important health services (e.g., Fig. 8). Disparities in usage of preventive health services exist for children as in Fig. 9 and adults (not shown); those with lower family income are far less likely to use preventive health services. Racial and ethnic minorities are also less likely to have a primary care clinician as a usual source of care (Fig. 10).

Perhaps most concerning are the health-care disparities. Examples of care disparities are displayed in Figs. 11, 12, and 13. In Fig. 11, there is a clear difference such that those with lower levels of education are less likely to report good communication with their health-care providers. Persons with higher levels of disability are also less likely to report that their health-care provider gives instructions that are easy to understand (Fig. 12). The disparities gap displayed in Fig. 13 is simply heartbreaking. Persons with lower levels of education are more likely to report thinking that their health-care providers do not respect them.

Health Disparities and Cultural Competency

Cultural competency is related to health disparities but is distinctly different. Many medical and educational intuitions have embraced education modules to educate staff and students about the importance of being aware of and respectful toward the cultural differences between individuals in the medical and educational environments, including patients, providers, ancillary staff, and even students. Cultural competency is a way of being that is sensitive to differences in culture among individuals (even when they share some cultural similarities—perhaps they're both American—but also different, say an African American and an African Immigrant).

This is not an end-point driven concept, as in "I am certified culturally competent," but is instead a process of continuous learning and adapting to different people so that one may effectively work with others from a variety of different backgrounds (Lawless et al. 2014). Learning about health disparities can support one being culturally competent, and vice versa, as different cultures and backgrounds experience health disparities at different rates, and those disparities can be driven by culture (e.g., diet, exercise, or alcohol consumption) or drive a cultural response (e.g., Tuskegee experiments leading to distrust of physicians in the African American community). Reading and reflecting on the narratives in this book is not expected to somehow cultivate cultural competence. Instead, a careful reading and thoughtful reflection can be best thought of as a starting point of cultural and narrative humility.

Intersecting Disparities

When studying health disparities, it is useful to consider the theory of intersectionality, first highlighted by civil rights advocate and legal scholar Kimberlé Williams Crenshaw, which considers how different identities can overlap and compound to influence an individual's experience of discrimination, oppression, and yes—even health disparities (Crenshaw 1989)! So what does that mean, exactly? Well, you cannot separate the woman from the African American from the lesbian or from the poverty. Each one of these traits, these identities, are inextricably linked and shape how this woman interacts with the world. One important part of intersectionality is to remember that these traits are not additive—it is not "woman + African American + lesbian + poor." Intersectionality theory instead highlights how these traits weave a complicated web that is not simply a stacking of identity like addition, but a multiplication of different interactive identities that have impacts on an individual relative to how society views and treats each identity held by a person.

It is easy to make assumptions about identities, but intersectionality allows for a deeper examination of the complex roles we all embody. For example, one might assume that, due to health disparities, white men have a consistent advantage over poor black women, however, research by medical sociologist Dr. Susan Hinze has shown that in American society, relatively "high power" wealthy, well-educated white men have similar levels of depression as relatively "low power" poor, low-education, black women, when compared to other members of society (Hinze et al. 2012).

As you read the narratives in this book, consider the intersections of the different identities for the patients *and* the providers. How do the identities come together for a man, who is also older, heterosexual, married, well-educated, and middle class? How would his experience be different if he held different identities? Would it change if he was white, gay, young, or poorly educated?

References

American Academy of Family Physicians (2018). Social determinants of health policy. http://www.aafp.org/about/policies/all/social-determinants.html. Accessed 6 Mar 2018

Crawford C (2018) The EveryONE project unveils social determinants of health tools. American Association of Family Physicians. https://www.aafp.org/news/health-of-the-public/20180109sdohtools.html. Accessed 31 Aug 2018

Crenshaw K (1989) Demarginalizing the intersection of race and sex: a black feminist critique of antidiscrimination doctrine, feminist theory and antiracist politics. U Chi Legal F 140:139–168

Healthy People 2020 (2018a) Disparities.https://www.healthypeople.gov/2020/about/foundation-health-measures/Disparities. Accessed 31 Aug 2018

Healthy People 2020 (2018b) Social determinants of health. https://www.healthypeople.gov/2020/topics-objectives/topic/social-determinants-of-health. Accessed 31 Aug 2018

Hinze SW, Lin J, Andersson T (2012) Can we capture the intersections? Older black women, education and health. Womens Health Issues 22:91–98

Lawless ME, Muellner J, Sehgal AR, Thomas CL, Perzynski AT (2014) Cultural competency education for researchers: a pilot study using a neighborhood visit approach. SOCRA Source 81:12–21

Orgera K, Artiga S (2018) Disparities in Health and Health Care: Five Key Questions and Answers. Kaiser Family Foundation https://www.kff.org/disparities-policy/issue-brief/disparities-in-health-and-health-care-five-key-questions-and-answers/. Accessed 31 Aug 2018

Names, events and details have been changed to protect privacy

Case Narratives

Adam Perzynski

A Note on How to Approach the Narratives in This Volume

As you pen your own narrative or read those contained in this text, consider what your first impression of these patients might be. What would be your visceral snap judgment of the situation? Next, let go of that first impression, and take a moment to more deeply ponder and unpack what you think of the patient in relation to her/his race, sexual orientation, gender, socioeconomic status, language barriers, or disability.

How is this person different from you? How are you alike? What challenges may she/he be facing because of health disparities? How may these differences impact the way someone trusts you or communicates with you?

Finally, consider other similar cases you've encountered previously. Are there any major differences, and/or are there any shared lessons that may help you address the social needs facing the patient in the case narrative?

A. Perzynski (✉)
Center for Health Care Research and Policy, The MetroHealth System, Case Western Reserve University, Cleveland, OH, USA
e-mail: Adam.Perzynski@case.edu

Part I
LBGT

Time to Leave

Ifeolorunbode Adebambo

This case narrative tells the story of a patient in words she would have used. Dr. B. is the physician recounting her patient's story and is the author of this narrative. The story is written in the first person to help the reader connect with the patient. The objective of sharing this case is to promote dialogue and understanding about the many diverse circumstances of persons who use health services.

I am an African American woman in her 40s who lives in the inner city and have been told I need a doctor to take care of my health needs. I want a woman of color and I found a doctor in the local safety net hospital. I discovered that she is a recent immigrant of African descent. I see that she supervises younger doctors in the Family Medicine office and has many patients.

The world has not been kind to me. I know I need medical care, but I am frustrated by the way I am being forced to conform to "what is" rather than be able to find what I want within the medical system that routinely discriminates and experiments on people of color. I need to stay strong or I will get swallowed up in the abyss of discrimination that is commonly encountered by women of color.

I hope my doctor of color is someone that I can relate to and speak with. I cannot stand the condescending tones and arrogance of the health-care system and those they try and force me to deal with. I do not want to be touched by anyone except someone of color and a female. They do not have a nurse of color here, and I refuse to deal with anyone not of color. Only Rose can take my vitals and draw my blood.

Feminism is the true religion, and mother earth is my strength. When I think of God, I know God is female. Our society portrays God as male, which is in keeping with the oppression they want to keep us under.

I keep my dark glasses on so that they do not know what I am thinking, but I can observe them. I know about my health and read widely. Contrary to thoughts about people of color, I am health literate. I prefer to use alternative therapies such as herbs and supplements rather than medications. At least there is no record that those have been used to experiment on people of color.

I. Adebambo (✉)
Department of Family Medicine, The MetroHealth System, Cleveland, OH, USA
e-mail: badebambo@metrohealth.org

© The Author(s) 2019
A. Perzynski et al. (eds.), *Health Disparities*,
https://doi.org/10.1007/978-3-030-12771-8_4

21

My doctor cares. She tries to accommodate me, I know, but a lot she asks I cannot do. A pelvic exam is impossible. I have never been able to tell anyone how I was raped as a child and how I cannot have anything to do with men. Even my twin sister, the closest person to me, doesn't know this. I needed to tell someone about this and told only my doctor. She suggested an exam under anesthesia. That scares me even more but I cannot show it. I am a strong woman of color.

I let her do a pap smear today since she keeps bothering me, just to make her happy. I still don't think I need one as I only have female partners. She insists though, tells me there is still a risk, and I have decided to trust her. I could not relax; she was very patient, but the test was very uncomfortable. I think I knew deep down it would lead to other issues. The result comes back abnormal. She wants me to get a colposcopy—I struggle to pronounce it. It is when they take samples of the neck of my womb. With *another* doctor. She has set it up and will come with me if I want her to.

I went for the test by myself, and this time it was not uncomfortable; it was $#@ @##% painful and guess what? More abnormality and I now need treatment. I will only see a woman of color. My doctor called five different hospitals and no fu$$$$$$#### woman of color anywhere to do this procedure. I will try the lady my younger sister sees on the other side of the city though she is white.

Three Years Later

I'm back at my doctor's. I did not go for further tests like I said I would and did not want to come back to my doctor. I'm back because my twin sister has kidney failure from untreated diabetes, and she made me swear to see a doctor. My sister is standing outside to make sure I come in. Dr. B. is the only doctor I will see.

The doctor does a pelvic exam. I am unable to tolerate a speculum exam and she abandons the procedure. After the finger exam I can tell there is something wrong. She tells me my cervix feels hard and that I have may have cervical cancer, but she cannot tell for sure till I get a biopsy. She begs me to see a GYN doctor and would refer me to a gentle humane doctor of Asian descent which I find more acceptable. She offers to talk to any family member or friend of my choice if I would like. I know she wants to tell my sister but I refuse. She is going through enough. I need to be strong for her. I already feel guilty that she is ill and I am not.

I saw the gynecologist and agreed to an examination under anesthesia. The biopsies show that I have cervical cancer. I think the biopsies are false. This is just another way to deceive people of color. I do not believe I have cancer. I trust my doctor but she trusts the system too much. I want a second opinion.

It took me 6 weeks to get a second opinion. My doctor has been calling me almost every week. They agree with the initial diagnosis but what do I expect within the same system? Anyway, regardless of their findings, I do not find any of the treatment options offered such as surgery or radiation acceptable.

When I was admitted the last time, I would only deal with the resident of color. My doctor had to come up every day to see me. The other doctor is familiar with the lesbian/gay community and suggested a healer. I agree to work with the healer. We got on well, and she was helpful for a few months but then also started to try and get me to consider treatment. We do not talk anymore.

My family sees my point of view. They know my doctor is from a rich African country and cannot understand my position. They stand with my decision. Only my younger sister is pushing me to get treatment, and she is extremely angry with my twin sister and me. I cannot talk to her and will continue to ignore her.

I am depressed; there is so much going on. My twin sister has been very ill recently. I'm under a lot of different pressures from my family, and my partner and I are no longer together. Dr. B. has suggested a psychiatrist of color—they have two. One is not taking new patients and the other I'll ask my sister to see. If I like her after my sister's visit, I will make an appointment with her. I did not like her, and I found the whole experience traumatic. I'll never go back again.

I missed my last appointment with my doctor. At my request, she printed at least 50 pages of information for me and my family. I have not changed my mind; I still refuse to go through any treatment.

I'm in a lot of pain, the vaginal odor is upsetting. I have been in hospital three times. I know the nurses and social workers hate me but right now I don't care. They need to do their jobs. Dr. B. convinces me to speak to the radiation oncologist who is a man of color. I will try and go.

After my last admission into hospital, I cannot take care of myself anymore. I choose to go to a nursing home. Dr. B. comes to visit me in the nursing home and tries to make sure I am comfortable. I'm dying and we all know it. My sister is angry with my doctor for not making me obey her recommendations. I think she is just frustrated with everything. Nobody can make me. I have told her to leave Dr. B. alone.

I hate the health-care system that forces me to refuse treatment. I admire Dr. B. for being able to function in this system however difficult, and I told her so. It is time for me to leave.

How Can We Care for Everyone?

Christina Antenucci

When I first met Charlotte, she was a 15-year-old African American boy named John.

I was a white physician working at a community health center in one of the poorest zip codes in Cleveland. John and her mother came in for a well-child exam to get vaccines and complete forms for school. As with all my teenage patients, I talked briefly with John alone to screen for high-risk health behaviors. John disclosed that she had unprotected sex with males, so I gave her condoms and encouraged safe sex. I also told her about confidential minor visits, where she had the option to see me without a parent to address her sexual health issues. After that, John usually came to see me without her mom.

John would come in to get tested for infections, get more condoms, and just talk. Her mother and brother knew about her being homosexual, but John felt isolated in her school and community. She connected with an LGBT teen group in downtown Cleveland for support. And she kept coming to see me.

As John became an adult, she started wearing makeup and jewelry. She began calling herself Charlotte and talked of gender reassignment surgery. She "borrowed" hormones from her friends. My medical assistants sometimes got confused when putting her in a room to be seen. Her medical records said "male" named "John," but she looked like a "female" named "Charlotte." Sometimes the wrong papers were in her file. I tried to alter the electronic record to reflect her female identity and avoid future confusion, but the software system did not accommodate such a change at that time. This was years before the current transgender movement, and much of the existing health-care system was not ready for Charlotte. Including me.

C. Antenucci (✉)
MetroHealth Family Medicine Residency, Cleveland, OH, USA

Case Western Reserve University School of Medicine, Cleveland, OH, USA

NEOMED, Rootstown, OH, USA
e-mail: cantenucci@metrohealth.org

© The Author(s) 2019
A. Perzynski et al. (eds.), *Health Disparities*,
https://doi.org/10.1007/978-3-030-12771-8_5

I was ignorant on the topic of transgender medical care. I had lesbian and gay patients, but this was my first patient who needed gender reassignment surgery. I read to educate myself on the basics. I found doctors who could help with her gender transition, but the clinic was across town. I arranged transportation to the LGBT PRIDE clinic at our hospital for evaluation and hormone therapy. She went a few times but then stopped going. She kept coming to see me. My clinic was closer, and we knew each other.

One week, Charlotte called me about a red eye and headache. I asked her to come see me, but she couldn't come in. So, I gave her ibuprofen and told her to rest. She called a week later with the same complaint. I insisted she come to see me. When she walked into my office, I was shocked. Her left eye was swollen, red, weeping, and partially bulging out of its socket. How was it possible that no one had taken her to an emergency room? Who looked at her each day? Should I have seen her sooner? I had an ambulance take her to the main hospital where she had a brain scan and surgery that night to drain an abscess. After weeks of antibiotics, Charlotte came back to see me. But she was different. Confused. Forgetful. Her appointments were more sporadic. And then I moved to a different clinic farther from her neighborhood, and we lost touch.

I often think of Charlotte and wonder how she is managing. Is she alive? Was she able to recover her cognitive functioning? Did she get her gender reassignment surgery? I feel anger at our society's failure to care for the most vulnerable. Where was the village helping raise this child? The family, the teachers, the church, the neighbors? And what of the doctor? What health-care system would have given this story a better ending?

Part II
Race, Ethnicity and Culture

Where Is the Patient? Finding the Person in Patient-Centered Health Care

Adam Perzynski, Carol Blixen, and Martha Sajatovic

MR. GREEN: I told my wife to bring my clothes. I dressed in my clothes and I was ready to go. Well it was kind of, it was kind of hilarious. I was just preparing myself to go home. So I dressed in my suit 1 day, and I really realized, that's how it really hit me, that the nurses and doctors didn't know me because I was sitting in the room and they were looking for me. And I was in my shirt and tie and everything.

[Laughter]

MR. GREEN: And that really, really they were looking…

MRS. GREEN: They were looking for somebody in the gown.

MR. GREEN: It really hit me because it's just sitting here I'm a number here. And it really, and I kept thinking about, I'm just a number. I sit there for 45 minutes and the doctors didn't really know me. And I sat there in the room there and they kept coming in, and I said these nurses don't know me.

MRS. GREEN: They thought you were a visitor.

MR. GREEN: They thought I was a visitor.

[Laughter]

MR. GREEN: The doctors came in and talked all around me, they talked and looking for me. I said, [to myself] "They don't know me. They don't even. They just know me as a patient," and I sat there in the room in the corner. I just sat there listening and looking and they was talking, "Where did he go?"

MR. GREEN: So they started looking for me on the floor. I said, [to myself] "They don't have no contact with me, they just came to service me." Even the lady that

A. Perzynski
Center for Health Care Research and Policy, The MetroHealth System, Case Western Reserve University, Cleveland, OH, USA

C. Blixen
Case Western Reserve University, Neurological and Behavioral Outcomes Center, University Hospitals, Cleveland Medical Center, Cleveland, OH, USA

M. Sajatovic (✉)
University Hospitals Cleveland Medical Center Case Western Reserve University School of Medicine, Cleveland, OH, USA
e-mail: martha.sajatovic@uhhospitals.org

© The Author(s) 2019
A. Perzynski et al. (eds.), *Health Disparities*,
https://doi.org/10.1007/978-3-030-12771-8_6

29

brought my breakfast. They stood there and I sat there and I watched. It was like a movie, and I'm watching. I was there, and I did that on the seventh day.

MR. GREEN: So on the seventh day they don't know me, and I said well maybe they have a lot of patients.

FACILITATOR: Did that make you feel less confident in your medical team?

MR. GREEN: I didn't think of it that way. It told me I need to get the heck on out of here.

[Laughter]

MR. GREEN: And I said I need to get the heck on out of here. Because I know they need, they have a lot of patients. I said I need to get the heck on out of here. People know who I am. They didn't even, and I watched this like I was on camera.

FACILITATOR: And they never even acknowledged you sitting there?

MRS. GREEN: No, not until I came. And I said this, "Are you looking for my husband? He's right here."

MR. BROWN: But they saw you sitting there, they saw you?

MRS. GREEN: Yeah they saw.

MR. BROWN: Did they ever say well, why are you here? Or what are you doing here?

MR. GREEN: No.

MRS. GREEN: They were looking for the patient.

MR. GREEN: They were looking for the patient cause I was in my…

MRS. GREEN: Cause he was in a suit.

MR. BROWN: Well I mean the reason I'm asking, you were in the patient's room.

MR. GREEN: I was in my room.

MR. BROWN: I would have thought they would have asked you well why are you?

MRS. GREEN: Yes, where did he go? Who are you? Well where is he?

MR. GREEN: Nothing.

MR. GREEN: They didn't ask you anything?

MRS. GREEN: Nothing.

MR. GREEN: I got up that morning, I shaved, everything the whole nine yards. Got ready, put my clothes on and this went on and I watched it.

MR. BROWN: But they did see you sitting there.

MRS. GREEN: Oh yeah. Yes, but they didn't acknowledge him, honey.

MR. GREEN: They saw me there. When I acknowledged it, I saw the reaction and it was angry, because one of the things that I discovered because they had other patients and I put them behind their schedule, looking for me.

MR. GREEN: And once their schedule was off, they didn't treat me the same way. They were very upset. Non-verbal communication shown, you know. They were very upset. It had a great impact because I said [to myself], "I can't be here because they don't know me," and they weren't trying to know me. They were doing a job, a service job to get me well, but I know they had a lot of patients, but they don't really know me.

MR. GREEN: So when I left that day and that just really, I didn't leave until 9:00 that night. They had me scheduled to leave, but I thought maybe they were penalizing me. We were sitting off to leave since 11:00 that morning. And I didn't get released until 9:00 that night. So I felt, I hope they weren't penalizing me.

MR. GREEN: But I didn't say anything. I just said when I get home I won't do that again.

Unacceptable

Hongfei Di

A Chinese speaking, middle-aged male patient shows up in my outpatient office, frustrated, and yet relieved to see me, as I am like him, also Chinese. The man started the encounter by complaining about the care provided by the "lao wai" doctors, which means foreign doctors. He stated that he was seen in the emergency department (ED) twice for chest palpitations and that he was not given a correct diagnosis. I immediately decided to look into the matter with some hope of resolving any possible confusion or misdiagnosis. After chart review, I was able to see that our ED managed him very well and performed examinations and tests to rule out acute coronary syndrome on two different occasions when this man visited the ED. The patient stated that the emergency physicians were unable to explain his palpitations, because they didn't care about Chinese people, and he further stated that they judged him because he spoke poor English. As I sat there explaining all of the tests and procedures that were done, I wondered if he had a legitimate reason to have this kind of thought process. I was not there during his visit to the emergency room and could not know how he had been treated by the care team.

Throughout the rest of the visit, I was able to dive deeper into the root of his palpitations. As it turns out, he had discovered his best friend dead in his apartment a few weeks ago, prior to the onset of his symptoms. He relayed the story, "He was my age, he had a family like me, I do not understand how he passed so suddenly." He further informed me that he had experienced similar symptoms many years ago in China when another friend of his was hit by a car in front of him and died. My doubt of cardiogenic etiologies increased.

As I began to explain his symptoms are likely rooted to psychogenic etiology, this patient became extremely defensive and upset, stating that I was labeling him a mental patient, that he is not crazy. As I tried to redirect and further explain, he further stated that Chinese men are healthy in the mind, and all the men in his family are great providers and none of them was ever crazy or sent to a mental institution

H. Di (✉)
Cleveland Clinic, Cleveland, OH, USA

© The Author(s) 2019
A. Perzynski et al. (eds.), *Health Disparities*,
https://doi.org/10.1007/978-3-030-12771-8_7

and he will most certainly not be the first. Further reiterating that he has heart issues, he refused to hear any more of my explanation and ultimately rejected my medication suggestions, which were in line with his anxiety symptoms. This man who was initially relieved to see me, refused to see me again and now concluded he would rather go to the ED for further care, informing me that I was worse than the "lao wai" doctors.

Testing Trust

Oluwatoyin Vivian Opelami

Mr. H is a 70-year-old African American man who walked into my office to establish care with me. His previous primary care physician had recently retired. I see him at a neighborhood primary care clinic that primarily serves African Americans. He is a polite, well-dressed gentleman with a high school education. Mr. H's first visit with me went well, but he had an unresolved complaint that had been going on for several months. He had complained of generalized burning pain that bothered him most of the day. He could not recall an inciting event and had not been able to find relief with previous therapies.

During the course of our discussion, I asked if he had ever been evaluated or treated for a sexually transmitted disease (STD), including syphilis. He denied ever having had an STD since he had been in a monogamous relationship for a long time, with his wife of more than 40 years. Towards the end of the visit, we discussed the plan of care and I indicated that tertiary syphilis was a possible cause of neuropathic pain and that screening for syphilis should be considered in addition to other tests such as vitamin B12 and folic acid levels.

However, I noticed a change in his demeanor as he looked disturbed. I asked him what the problem was and his reply was quite shocking to me. He informed me of some acquaintances who had been infected with syphilis in Tuskegee, Alabama, where he was from and wondered if that could have happened to him. There was a long pause where I was unable to find an appropriate response to his question. I advised him to take some time to decide if he wanted to find out and to come back whenever he was ready.

I guess I got "schooled" that day on sensitivity to the plight of African Americans as it pertains to historical issues. I inquired among the nursing and medical assistant staff of the clinic about Tuskegee, and they explained to me the history of the

O. V. Opelami (✉)
School of Medicine, Case Western Reserve University and The MetroHealth System,
Cleveland, OH, USA
e-mail: oopelami@metrohealth.org

© The Author(s) 2019
A. Perzynski et al. (eds.), *Health Disparities*,
https://doi.org/10.1007/978-3-030-12771-8_8

U.S. Public Health Service Syphilis Study at Tuskegee, and how hundreds of African American men with syphilis were not offered penicillin despite its availability after 1947. As a recent immigrant to the United States and an African-trained physician myself, I suddenly realized the impact of prior historical issues on a patient's perceptions and acceptance of my recommendations. The social and emotional wounds of the Tuskegee study are real and are still being felt by families as far away as Cleveland, Ohio, more than 15 years after the last participant in the study died and more than 50 years after the study officially ended in 1972.

A few weeks after his initial visit, Mr. H returned to the office with his wife to discuss the possibility of getting screened for syphilis. We had a long discussion on the effects of tertiary syphilis on the nervous system, the possibility of these effects being permanent and available treatment options. The test was done and he was referred to neurology for the ongoing pain issue. Unfortunately, I have not seen him since that last visit. I am unsure if this was due to the emotional impact of his visits with me or a distrust of the health-care system in general.

The System is Unfair

Wisler Saint-Vil

45-year-old African American male with medical history significant for chronic low back pain, spinal stenosis s/p laminectomy 2012, HTN, CKD stage V on dialysis. No history of illicit drug use, drinks alcohol occasionally, doesn't smoke.

I saw that patient once in the clinic and took care of him for 4 days when he was admitted for community acquired pneumonia. Patient has been complaining of his PCP not willing to prescribe him stronger pain medication. The Tylenol he is taking doesn't really relieve the pain. He has tried physical therapy multiple times which doesn't help with the pain. Since the laminectomy, the low back pain has been worse. He thinks that his PCP has been refusing to give him stronger pain medication because he is black. He thinks that doesn't make any sense because he doesn't have a history of illicit drug abuse, not even a smoker. He would like to switch PCP, his actual PCP is white, and he thinks if he has a PCP of color, maybe she/he can treat him better.

The patient also complained of the health-care system to be unfair. Since he is young, he was thinking about getting a kidney transplant from organ donation. He asked his nephrologist who proceeded to inform him that he is doubtful he will ever have a kidney donation that will match, because he is black and black people don't usually donate organs. This was offered as an explanation of why they tend to favor white patients who are in the waiting list. The patient told me that he is very confused. He can't understand how the health-care system is that unfair.

W. Saint-Vil (✉)
MetroHealth Medical Center, Cleveland, OH, USA
e-mail: wsaintvil@metrohealth.org

© The Author(s) 2019
A. Perzynski et al. (eds.), *Health Disparities*,
https://doi.org/10.1007/978-3-030-12771-8_9

Part III
Gender

The Irritable Uterus

Rebecca Fischbein

The patient was a 33-year-old, highly educated, white female. She was pregnant with monochorionic-diamniotic identical twins, or twins that shared the same placenta but were in separate amniotic sacs. She had been cleared from her reproductive endocrinologist at 13 weeks gestation after an ultrasound indicated the pregnancy was progressing typically. The patient was referred back to her primary obstetrician, along with her pregnancy records, for the remainder of her prenatal care. She had multiple appointments over the next few weeks during which the fetuses' heartbeats were examined. The patient mentioned she was having some periodic, light contractions but otherwise all was normal.

At approximately 18 weeks gestation, after calling her obstetrician for persistent, painless contractions, she was told to go immediately to the emergency room (ER). She was asked to provide a urine sample to test for infection, which returned negative. She was given intravenous (IV) fluids for hydration. No additional exams or tests were conducted, and she was released. The following week, she was again referred to the ER as the contractions had continued and become much more frequent, and she was now extremely uncomfortable and very worried. She was presenting with approximately 30 low-intensity contractions per minute. Her urine tested negative for infection and she was given an IV for hydration. She was given a fetal fibronectin test which was also negative. No additional tests or exams were conducted. She was given the diagnosis of uterine irritability and released. She had a follow-up appointment 2 days later at her primary obstetrician who confirmed the diagnosis. No additional tests were conducted or instructions provided.

The patient continued to feel extensive discomfort and concern over the next week and decided to remain in bed or sitting as those positions were the most comfortable. She returned to her primary obstetrician's practice for her previously

R. Fischbein (✉)
Department of Family and Community Medicine, Northeast Ohio Medical University,
Rootstown, OH, USA
e-mail: rfischbein@neomed.edu

© The Author(s) 2019
A. Perzynski et al. (eds.), *Health Disparities*,
https://doi.org/10.1007/978-3-030-12771-8_10

scheduled 20-week ultrasound. The ultrasound technician found the first fetus and determined it was female. The technician and the patient noted the fetus was floating in excessive amounts of amniotic fluid. The technician next found the other fetus and both the technician and the patient observed the other fetus was not moving; it appeared stuck to the wall of the uterus with no amniotic fluid. The technician informed the patient that the fetuses were likely suffering from twin-twin transfusion syndrome and quickly informed the doctor on duty. The patient was told by the physician she had a severe case of the syndrome and would require immediate referral and treatment. She was further informed it was likely that she would lose at least one fetus. Due to the excess of fluid around the one fetus, her abdomen was measuring at 28 weeks even though she was only 20 weeks. The patient suspected immediately it was the effects of this syndrome that she had been feeling for weeks. Yet, in the many times she had been to her obstetrician and ER, no one had listened to her concerns that something was very wrong. No one had thought to conduct an ultrasound to test her for this known risk of this pregnancy type.

That patient was me. After additional battles that included surgeries while pregnant and preterm labor, I had a happy ending concluding with two live births and babies who survived their time in the NICU. I chose to title this "The Irritable Uterus" because it reduces me and my experience to a female body part with a minor diagnosis, albeit an inaccurate one. This exemplifies how I felt during this time; I was simply a uterus that was irritable and was also irritating the healthcare professionals around me. I was annoying everyone by repeatedly sharing my concerns about what they thought was a seemingly normal symptom of twin pregnancies and, in response, those concerns were brushed off.

Barriers to the Breast

Sandra Wright-Esber

Jessica is a 22-year-old African American woman and just had her third baby. She is not married and has two other children and very little help at home. She works as a nurse's aide at a nursing home. No one in her family has breastfed, but she has heard it is a good thing for her baby. Jessica and the baby's dad recently broke up, but he wants to help as much as he can; he is not sure if breastfeeding is a good idea or not. She had trouble coming for prenatal care because she takes the bus (she does not have a car), so taking the free breastfeeding and childbirth education classes was more or less out of the question. Those classes are mostly at night. She had five prenatal visits and took her prenatal vitamins faithfully. She delivers a full-term, healthy baby girl who weighs 6 pounds 14 ounces. She has received and read a handout about breastfeeding at one prenatal visit from the nurse, and her OB told her breastfeeding is good for her baby. Right after delivery, she is given her baby to breastfeed and it goes well. The baby latches on and nurses on both breasts for about 30 minutes. She is so happy that the baby is healthy and that this labor and delivery was easier than her past two deliveries.

Once Jessica and the baby transfer to the postpartum floor, she is instructed by her nurse to breastfeed on demand, about every 2–3 hours. The next time the baby is awake, she tries to feed her, but the baby cries for 5 minutes and makes a few attempts to latch on but then falls asleep. She calls the nurse to help, and the nurse says she will be right there but is unable to come for about 30 minutes. The nurse apologizes and then shows the mom some ways to wake the baby up to feed and shows her how to latch the baby to the breast properly. The baby only tries to nurse for about 3 minutes and then falls asleep. It goes on like this for about six more hours with the baby nursing for a few minutes and then falling asleep for about 2 hours at a time.

S. Wright-Esber (✉)
The MetroHealth System, Cleveland, OH, USA
e-mail: sesber@metrohealth.org

© The Author(s) 2019
A. Perzynski et al. (eds.), *Health Disparities*,
https://doi.org/10.1007/978-3-030-12771-8_11

Jessica has not slept for about 20 hours when she was in labor and is now tired and it is late at night. The night shift nurse is worried that the mom looks exhausted and offers to take the baby to the nursery and assures the mom that she will feed her a bottle of formula if the mom agrees to that. She is very worried that her baby has not really eaten and is happy to think of getting a few hours sleep so she agrees. It has been a happy, exciting day. The baby receives two bottles of formula that night.

In the morning, I come to the Jessica's room to do the baby's first admission exam as the nurse practitioner covering the nursery. I do the exam in the room so the mom can watch and ask questions. The baby is very healthy and has a normal physical exam. I ask the mom how she wants to feed her baby, and she says she wants to breastfeed. We talk about the best ways to breastfeed, which include keeping the baby near skin-to-skin contact to promote frequent feedings and avoiding any formula or pacifiers as much as possible at least for the first 3 weeks, if not longer. Jessica tells me that the nurse gave two bottles last night and the baby seemed to like it.

I am supportive but tell her that to breastfeed successfully, it is important to get a good milk supply early and she needs to do that by nursing frequently and not offering formula. She listens to me but says it is hard to be the only one who can feed her baby; she is not sure she will be able to do this at home because she is busy with her two other children and work. She says she will think about what I have told her. I check on her the following day, and she has given six bottles of formula and has only breastfed twice. I am careful to support her choice; I know given the circumstances of keeping up with work, her two other children, and other difficulties, Jessica faces this challenge with fewer resources than many women.

The Annual Big Girl/Big Boy Exchange

Kristin Baughman

Several years ago, when I had a painful cyst on my ovary, my family doctor referred me to an OB/GYN. He is not the physician I would have chosen. I prefer female doctors, but I was anxious to get care quickly, and the physician seemed knowledgeable and willing to discuss options with me, so I stuck with him for future yearly exams. I did not want to seem sexist by insisting on a female physician.

Sometime in my 40s, the US Preventive Services Task Force (USPSTF) came out with new guidelines for the timing of mammograms for women my age: every other year rather than every year. When the doctor wrote a prescription for my yearly mammogram, I told him that I would like to skip a year. He responded incredulously, "well you are a big girl now, so I will let you make that decision," along with a lecture about the importance of early screening. A "big girl?" and "let" me make that decision? Is that what he would have said to a male patient refusing a PSA test? "Well, you are a big boy now…" I wanted to scream that I was a professor teaching evidence-based medicine, and I knew the current recommendations and understood screening exams, the risk of false positives, and the difference between soft and hard outcome measures. Did he? But I kept my mouth shut, smiled, and left. I did not get a mammogram to his dismay.

A couple of years later at one of my annual exams, he noticed that I had gone off my birth control pills and wondered what I was using. Given his patronizing attitude in the past, I was reluctant to tell him that I no longer needed birth control because I was dating a woman. Knowing that I had the power and the health insurance to switch doctors at any time, I decided humor was the best approach, "I'm using Kathy." He looked puzzled so I explained that I had switched from a male partner to a female partner. He smiled and said, "sounds like a Seinfeld episode—you're batting for the other team, now." Thank god. No patronizing or homophobic comments, just some comic relief. The next year when he performed surgery on me, he treated

K. Baughman (✉)
Northeast Ohio Medical University, Rootstown, OH, USA
e-mail: kbaughma@neomed.edu

Kathy with the utmost respect as my significant other and kept her informed of every step. The guy did have a heart: a patronizing heart, but a heart nonetheless.

Last year the USPSTF recommendations for mammograms changed once again. They recommended that women in their 50s could also limit mammograms to every other year so I skipped another year. When my doctor asked if I had received a mammogram last year, I told him, "No, I skipped last year." Back was the condescending comment about being a "big girl" so he would "let" me make that decision. Once again I smiled and left.

I feel like I should speak up and tell him that I don't appreciate being called a "girl." If I don't speak up, will anyone else feel empowered to speak up? He knows that I am a highly educated professor at the medical school. If he is patronizing toward me, how does he treat his patients with less education or resources? Is he even more patronizing toward them? Does he let them make decisions? More importantly, does he give them the tools they need to make their own informed decisions? My guilt from ignoring the comments weighs on my conscience. It is easier to just smile, ignore the comment, and take the easy route. After all, I was trained well as a woman to smile and move on. But that feminist professor inside me wants to put him in his place. Now that he is a "big boy," he needs a lesson in evidence-based medicine and respect for women.

Part IV
Poverty

I Hurt Everywhere

David Sperling

Dr. S: Diffuse pain, possible drug-seeking behavior.

Ms. K: *Doc, I hurt everywhere. I've had all kinds of tests and no one can figure out what's wrong with me. I went to the ER again last week because my chest was hurting and I was afraid it was my heart. They said it wasn't my heart and I need to see a PCP.*

Dr. S: A 32-year-old African American female, first visit, non-specific pain complaints (These visits feel more like a battle than a collaboration.)

Ms. K: *Every part of my body hurts, I can't sleep, I can't remember the last time I felt good and the medicine they gave me at the ER doesn't make me feel better at all.*

Dr. S: Complaint of daily symptoms for years. Also, complaint of insomnia. No relief with multiple NSAIDs and muscle relaxers prescribed during multiple ER visits (Here comes the request for pain meds.)

Ms. K: *I've had to call off work as a dishwasher because my arms, legs, and back hurt, and I can't stand at the sink washing because of the pain. My boss says if I call off again I will be fired.*

Dr. S: Difficulty with some ADLs and work as a result of symptoms (Here comes the request for disability!)

Ms. K: *I have to take the bus to Mississippi in a few days. My mother's brother was shot and I want to be there with my family for the funeral. When I sit for a long time I feel even worse. Can you give me something so I will be able to sit for 18 h on the greyhound?*

Dr. S: (I knew it!) Tell you what, let's do a physical exam.

Dr. S: Depressed, anxious-appearing African American female.

D. Sperling (✉)
Department of Family and Community Medicine, Northeast Ohio Medical University,
Rootstown, OH, USA
e-mail: dsperling@neomed.edu

© The Author(s) 2019
A. Perzynski et al. (eds.), *Health Disparities*,
https://doi.org/10.1007/978-3-030-12771-8_13

Dr. S: Diffuse tender points to light palpation in periarticular regions in upper and lower extremities, back and neck.

Ms. K: *Damn doc, it HURTS when you push there.*

Dr. S: Exam otherwise unremarkable.

Dr. S: Fibromyalgia.

Ms. K: *I don't know what fancy name you are calling it. All I know is that I feel bad, I hurt everywhere, and I can't remember a time when I felt good. Doctors just tell me what it isn't but they never tell me what it is. I can't do my job feeling like this. I need relief!*

Dr. S: Suggest trial of tricylic antidepressant as indicated for fibromyalgia.

Ms. K: *Doc, I ain't depressed. Why are you giving me those depression pills? I need something for these PAINS.*

Dr. S: Regular aerobic exercise.

Ms. K: *Doc, I don't have a gym I can go to for aerobics. I can't walk in my neighborhood without getting mugged or shot and there are no sidewalks. Even if it was safe, I'd have to walk in the street.*

Dr. S: Sleep hygiene.

Ms. K: *Doc, I am not a dirty person. Just because I'm poor doesn't mean I don't take care of my hygiene!*

Waiting

Mary Corrigan

The schedule was full and the patients were stacked back-to-back every 20 minutes. Not bad for a general practice, but with wheelchairs, gurneys, and slow tortoise-like strides of the confused meandering into the unfamiliar, it may as well have been 5-minute visits. The onerous check-in, endless validation of insurance cards, and collection of co-pays with the subsequent querying of medications and *concerns of others*—the goal at the end being to share with **your** doctor **your** concerns is truncated and rushed. This is only magnified by the patient who repeatedly "no-shows" and has now arrived 40 minutes late. The factory line has been disrupted; the conveyor belt is broken. It starts with the front office staff wondering and going up the chain of command; "Should we reschedule?" "Can we fit them in?" "What is our policy?" "They have no showed 3 times in the past." "What is the patient's responsibility in all of this?"

The lunch break is near and once again nonexistent due to the clinic running over time. The ***chronic no-show*** and **now late** patient arrives to have **her** concerns addressed. Apologetic and flustered, the demoralized diabetic woman is chastised at the desk for her previous absences and current late arrival.

The visit occurs as many others do. The feet are checked, the blood sugar log is recorded, and the medications are reconciled. Laboratory tests are monitored, referrals are entered, and the patient is once again sent on her way for a repeat scenario in a couple of months. As the cycle does not get broken, the pattern does not change. The practitioner and patient are frustrated. The hemoglobin A1C is rarely within normal range, and the staff cringes when the name appears on the roster, knowing what they are in store for.

Finally, it is disclosed that the mislabeled patient has dutifully attempted to be compliant with her visits; the system has failed her. Her home is located 15 miles away, a 30-minute drive at best. Her journey is anything but straightforward.

M. Corrigan (✉)
Case Western Reserve University, The MetroHealth System, Cleveland, OH, USA
e-mail: mcorrigan@metrohealth.org

© The Author(s) 2019
A. Perzynski et al. (eds.), *Health Disparities*,
https://doi.org/10.1007/978-3-030-12771-8_14

She has been in a maze of thoroughfares and transit systems. She has been crafty in seeing through the miasma of her expedition. Waiting on the corner for the number 22 bus due at 8:05, it is now 8:15. Her route is then followed by a light rail "rapid transit" sojourn, rarely on time, followed by a transfer to the number 67 and a three-block walk to the finish line which creates a whole day's job to do that she knows is best for her own care. Glad to have arrived at all, she is met by a frustrated face and congratulated only with criticism. She is labeled as noncompliant.

Just Give Me Narcan and Let Me Go

Ali Ali

One of my responsibilities as a resident physician in family medicine is to work at our health-care system's community opioid overdose education and naloxone distribution program. While sitting at the table with a colleague waiting for a patient to show up, this 19-year-old Caucasian female walked in and introduced herself and sat at the other side of the table.

"I want Narcan …" she said.

She looked so tired and was not maintaining an eye contact as if she feels ashamed.

"Why do you need Narcan?" I replied.

"Yesterday I witnessed a close friend of mine at a party collapsing and she was unable to breathe. I gave her Narcan and after few minutes, she woke up."

"I need Narcan because I am afraid that I will be like her one day and I will need help.

I don't want to die. I have been doing drugs all my life and I can't stop right now. I don't know where my parents are."

"Are you staying somewhere right now?" I asked, hoping to refer her to some other resources if needed.

"I just live with a couple of close friends that I know. We have been friends for a long time and we all use drugs. Give me the Narcan and let me go."

I took the Narcan out of the kit, completed the paperwork and asked her, "Do you know how to use it?"

She replied, "Yes I do, I saved my friend's life yesterday at the party and I know how to do CPR."

"Tell me about your medical history?"

"Well, I have kidney failure..."

"Do you have a doctor?"

A. Ali (✉)
Southern California Permanente Medical Group (SCPMG), Kern County,
Bakersfield, CA, USA

© The Author(s) 2019
A. Perzynski et al. (eds.), *Health Disparities*,
https://doi.org/10.1007/978-3-030-12771-8_15

"No."

"Why you don't go and see a doctor for your kidney failure?" I asked.

"I am afraid." She replied.

Worried for her, I asked, "Afraid of what?"

"Afraid of being captured or charged. I don't have insurance and I know they charge a lot of money in the hospital. I would rather lay on the ground and not breathe than go to the hospital."

I tried to talk to her and counsel her but she said again, "Just give the Narcan and let me go. That's how you will help me."

I gave her the Narcan. After she took it, on her way out, she turned back and said, "Doctor, I want to ask you a question."

"Of course, have a seat"

"Doctor, sometimes I get seizures, what do you think is causing it?"

For a moment, I was thinking how bad this young woman's situation is; she is coming today asking for help, being afraid of death after witnessing her friend almost die, and now she has all these medical conditions and questions that she hasn't been able to see a doctor for because of fear of being charged or captured. "Well, there are a lot of reasons why could someone have seizures. Were you ever been diagnosed with a seizure disorder?"

She explained, "I have never seen a doctor in my entire life."

"Can you come and see me in the clinic?"

"No, I can't. I don't want to go to the hospital. They will treat me like shit and I will be charged. I don't have money and I don't..." And she left the room.

It was such a heartbreaking moment to meet this young woman suffering in her life, addicted to drugs and unable to see a doctor to help her out, not only with addiction and her medical conditions but even just answering her questions. She was suffering more than she needed to due to barriers such as insurance, legal issues, and bias about the way these patients are being treated in the hospital that prevented her from seeking medical attention.

Part V
Inequality

New in Town

John Boltri

I finished my family medicine residency in June of 1990. I had been recruited by the vice chairman to join the faculty at the Department of Family and Community Medicine at the University of Texas Health Science Center in Houston but was not able to start until I acquired a Texas license. By the time the results of my board examination had been returned and I had passed the Texas medical jurisprudence exam, it was September. The Department was relatively large and hierarchical with a number of clinical sites. New faculty were expected to know how to practice and it was clear, or at least it appeared to be to me, that asking for help was not welcome. This was the first time I lived and worked south of the Mason-Dixon line and west of the Mississippi. That's a big deal because my Dean's letter specifically stated I would likely be practicing north of the Mason-Dixon line and east of the Mississippi, implying a decidedly Yankee background. Somehow the opposite happened and I spent 22 years in the south after growing up in the northeastern United States where I also completed my medical training.

So this story represents three patients with disparities from my earliest post-residency experience, a time filled with apprehension and anxiety, and the three patients in each story were all seen during the last few months of 1990. All three patients were born and raised Texans, a culture I had no knowledge of and for which I had little cultural competence.

Mrs. KS came to see me as a new patient to the practice. She had three children less than 10 years old and her husband of 10 years had recently died of AIDS. AIDS was discovered while I was a medical student and while effective treatments were emerging in the late 1980s and early 1990s, it was still considered by most of the public to be a fatal disease. On the other hand, because the treatment options were limited,

J. Boltri (✉)
Department of Family and Community Medicine, Northeast Ohio Medical University College of Medicine, Rootstown, OH, USA
e-mail: jboltri@neomed.edu

© The Author(s) 2019
A. Perzynski et al. (eds.), *Health Disparities*,
https://doi.org/10.1007/978-3-030-12771-8_16

many family physicians managed patients with HIV infection, and it was well known that aggressive treatment could extend life by 5 or maybe even 10 years or more.

Mrs. KS wanted to be tested for AIDS. We talked about HIV testing and follow-up. I don't remember much else about the first visit, but know I asked her a lot of questions about her deceased husband, her children, and support system because I had learned well during my residency training in family medicine that building a strong relationship with your patient was very important.

I do remember she was a woman shorter than myself (I am not a tall man) and quite thin. I don't recall if she was poor, while my memory tells me she was not well off, I do not specifically remember her being seriously resource deprived. I also recall she had unprotected intercourse with her husband throughout his illness. We did the testing she asked for and checked for STDs as well as some basic blood work. We agreed on a follow-up appointment in a week or two. Not surprisingly her HIV test was positive.

She came back for her follow-up appointment and I shared the news. This visit has stuck with me and is a recurrent memory. I explained the test results and informed her of the treatment options. I told her there were effective medications that could keep her healthy for a long time. She told me she was not interested in medication and that God would provide. I asked if we could talk about how she felt about the news and if I could talk about the therapy with her some more. She said no and got up to leave. I pleaded with her to stay and talk. She left and I never saw her again. Attempts to contact her were futile. When I think about that visit, I think about what I could have done differently. Starting from the first visit, getting to know her better, developing some shared values, anticipating the diagnosis, having a support person, and getting to know her culturally, spiritually and humanely. I always wonder what became of her and her children. I hope she found medical care elsewhere, but my heart tells me otherwise.

The next patient I saw during the same time-frame was also HIV+. He had been under the care of the department's vice-chair and was transferred to me shortly after I started working in the department. I no longer remember the vice-chair's reason for transferring the patient to my care, but I do remember not questioning the transfer. I had a few HIV+ patients and felt comfortable managing their care. This particular gentleman was a community service worker and had been doing well for about 1–1.5 years. At the first visit with me I discovered he had a few bouts of a recurrent perirectal abscess during the past few months. He was taking an antiviral agent five times a day as prescribed by my boss, the department vice-chair. This gentleman was about my age and well dressed in a nice button-down shirt and appeared to me to be very much like me. I sent him to a surgeon who drained the abscess under anesthesia. I also checked some blood tests, and the results showed a markedly low CD4 count – much lower than the two times it had been checked during the previous 12 months. That's when I scratched my head and asked him to return for another visit. Medication choices were limited, and if he wasn't controlled on his current regimen, that meant a referral to an infectious disease specialist and a strong possibility of a downward course – the beginning of the end so to speak.

At the return visit I confirmed that he was taking his medications five times a day without fail as he had been for the past 2 years. That's when I decided to take a deep dive into his life and learn everything about him. Born and raised in Houston, he was college educated and was happy with his life. He was gay and in a monogamous relationship. Coming out to his family had been difficult, but he was doing well. He was a cafeteria manager and worked long hours, often 12 hours a day, and was off on weekends. "How do you remember when to take your meds while you are working?" "Oh, I don't take the meds during the day." "Tell me more" I said. "Well it's hard to take them while I work. I don't want others to see me taking the meds." "I thought you told me you were taking them five times a day?" "I am." He was taking two in the morning about an hour apart and three in the evening about 2 hours apart. "Why are you doing it that way?" "Well, Dr. C said I could." Dr. C was my boss. "What did Dr. C tell you?" "He said I didn't have to take them exactly every four hours."

We found a way for him to take the meds every 4 hours while maintaining his dignity at work. His CD4 counts came up and infections cleared.

My last patient that sticks in my memory was a sweet older woman. I was 29 years old, she was only 59 but looked 70, thin and frail with wrinkled sun-damaged skin. She presented as a new patient with a complaint of foot pain. She walked a lot, sometimes all day and all night. She often walked from bar to bar at night and sometimes stopped but was usually not welcome. This past Saturday she had been walking for 3 hours without shoes on and had blisters on her feet. "Why three hours, why didn't you stop when your feet started hurting?" "I don't know. I couldn't stop." On history she had trouble with other things. She couldn't turn the lock an odd number of times or buy an odd number of things like one or three bars of soap, only an even number. This is a big problem if you are poor. Her weight was low. I don't remember her weight and I suspect her BMI was <20 but BMI was not something we routinely recorded in 1990. On exam she was thin and unkempt. Her hair was dirty and ungroomed, and she appeared to not have showered in at least a few days. She smelled of smoke from her cigarette use. She had blisters on both of her feet.

I knew from my training that she probably had obsessive compulsive disorder (OCD), but she had never been diagnosed or treated for that before. I asked her to come back in a few days and told her I would find out how we could best help her. Without insurance, I could not find a nearby psychiatrist to see her. Houston had a pretty good basic safety net, and after a few calls I was able to find a psychiatrist downtown who would see her. I scheduled a follow-up visit for 1 week. I wasn't sure if she was going to return to see me but she did. I had projected from her body language that she was indifferent. I told her I found someone for her to see and she seemed uninterested. She said she was hoping I would treat her. When I explained that we needed help, she still said she was not interested. My frustration was hard to hold back and she could tell. I explained that I really wanted to help her and would like to treat her as a patient, but in order to do that, she would also need to see a psychiatrist at least once. That's when she told me she has no way to get downtown. "What about the bus?" "I can't afford it" she said. Two dollars I thought. The round-trip was just a few packs of cigarettes - they were cheaper back then. I took out my wallet and gave her $2. She refused, I insisted. She left without saying thank you. I thought I would never see her again and was certain I had insulted her. I knew she was an uninsured person with no money, no resources, and most likely had obsessive compulsive disorder. I didn't understand her lifestyle, how she lived, what was important to her, or really anything about her but was certain I would never see her again.

She came back to see me the following month. Her hair was combed and she was well groomed. We had a routine office visit and she was doing very well. She had seen the psychiatrist and was taking medication. Her blisters had all healed and she was feeling good. We began to focus on preventive measures and scheduled a Pap and mammogram. On the way out she reached into her purse and handed me 20 dimes. This experience still brings tears to my eyes.

What I learned from these three experiences and what I continue to learn from my patients every day is that every person is different, forged by generations of relationships and experiences. All of these experiences fuse to shape every person differently with a set of beliefs and values that are different from my own, sometimes enormously different, and I can't even begin to understand a person and treat them with the utmost excellence unless I take the time to hear their story and understand who they are as a person in mind, body, and spirit. I, we, must listen to the patients and treat them all as fellow human beings honoring their values and wishes as best as possible.

Fleas

Vanessa H. Worley

A young man about the age of 14 came to the urgent care facility where I was working a late shift (4 pm to 9 pm) one evening. The teenager's mother accompanied him to the facility, and our front desk staff explained to her that we did not have the ability to evaluate his abdominal symptoms of diarrhea and vomiting, because often these require diagnostic tests that we cannot do at an urgent care center. She voiced understanding of the fact that the medical provider who saw her son that night may have to recommend the emergency department instead for more appropriate care. She voiced that she really just needed a note for his school to excuse his absence that related to his current illness. Their wait was long, as it was an especially busy evening. When I finally saw the patient in the exam room, I apologized for the long wait and thanked them for waiting. The mother explained that they could not leave because they *had* to get an excuse for his school; he was already in a special program after having excessive truancy and behavioral problems at his original school, and the requirements and consequences for absence now are very strict. The obese young man sat on the exam table and displayed a somewhat flat affect and low mood. He didn't make much eye contact and answered my questions softly and very briefly. When I had him lay down on the exam table to examine his abdomen, I noticed many, many black specks bouncing around on the white exam table paper moving in and out of the boy's black curly hair. Fortunately, his illness was a self-limited mild viral gastroenteritis that did not require any further treatment. I was able to provide them the school excuse saying that the boy had been seen and evaluated for illness on this day. The bigger part of my conversation with the boy and his mother that day centered around the fact that he had fleas and that they needed to treat him, their pets, and their entire home. It was an unexpected exam finding for

V. H. Worley (✉)
University of Mount Union, Alliance, OH, USA
e-mail: worleyvh@mountunion.edu

© The Author(s) 2019
A. Perzynski et al. (eds.), *Health Disparities*,
https://doi.org/10.1007/978-3-030-12771-8_17

me, the first time I saw this in the clinic. The mother seemed obviously embarrassed but also already aware of the problem because she was now requiring the cats to stay on the sun porch; she had not taken further steps. My heart broke for this young person whose health and future seemed to be so negatively and perhaps hopelessly impacted by the determinants in his life over which he had little to no control. The fleas seemed to be just the tip of the iceberg.

The Hungry Child and the Corner Store

Stacey Gardner-Buckshaw

Urban corner stores in Northeast Ohio have a reputation for contributing to neighborhood demise. Sales of liquor, cigarettes, lottery tickets, and other high-calorie low-nutrition foods along with high check-cashing fees have given corner stores titles such as "predatory" or "destructive."

However, neighborhood families have a very different view of the corner store. The corner store is also the only place local families without transportation can shop, and families are grateful to owners who keep the store in the neighborhood when all others have fled. It is a hangout for kids after school and for adults before and after work. While an urban corner store appears to be an unlikely partner to promote community health, it is a feasible location to reach the families in need.

The Community Action Agency where I worked recognized that families in Akron's Summit Lake neighborhood recognized the corner store owner as a leader. He was a young entrepreneur who had a successful business. As a result, we partnered with the neighborhood market/liquor store in an effort to promote community health. We provided the store with coolers, and in exchange the owner stocked fresh produce and supported the community garden across the street.

The issue of access to healthy food was surprisingly easy. Changing the culture of eating was much more difficult. Families without working appliances or any knowledge of food preparation were not eager consumers of garden-fresh produce.

In an effort to encourage the neighbors to try "new," healthy, low-cost foods, our agency started a "Taste It and Make It" series featuring produce carried by the store and produce from the community garden. The idea came from, now, Akron City Council Member At Large, Veronica Sims, in collaboration with the Summit Food Policy Coalition. Even though I was the Program Director, I decided I would be first to create my recipe and serve a healthy dish that I thought families would enjoy.

S. Gardner-Buckshaw, PhD, MPA (✉)
Department of Family and Community Medicine, Northeast Ohio Medical University, Rootstown, OH, USA
e-mail: sgardnerbuckshaw@neomed.edu

© The Author(s) 2019
A. Perzynski et al. (eds.), *Health Disparities*,
https://doi.org/10.1007/978-3-030-12771-8_18

I, with one of the agency community organizers, set up a display in a key area of the store – right in front of the liquor fridge. From 11 a.m. to 2 p.m. on a Tuesday in June, we introduced Italian pasta salad full of tomatoes, cucumbers, peppers, and olives to the neighbors. We surveyed the "tasters," asking them if they liked the pasta salad, and then gave them a recipe. For some new to shopping and cooking, we walked with them to the areas of the store where the ingredients could be purchased and then across the street to the garden where ingredients could be accessed at no cost. There were a few patrons that did not appreciate our presence in their hangout. However, most were happy to enjoy a free lunch and talked to us at great length about ways to eat healthier.

The part of the day that will stay with me forever was meeting a family of nine children. The mother/caretaker/aunt heard about the free meal and brought all of the kids. The mother was clearly coming down from a high and had not showered in quite some time. The kids, ranging in age from approximately 4 to 11 years and seemingly belonging to almost every local ethnic group, appeared to be well-kept. One young boy told me he had not eaten in several days. "Johnny" was 7, with blondish-brown hair and freckles. He was talkative, bright, and precocious. He asked many questions. "How do you get food? How do you find food if you don't have any money? How did you make the pasta salad? What is in pasta? Are kids allowed to eat at the summer lunch program if my aunt forgot to sign me up?"

I responded to the best of my ability, took the contact name of the caregiver, and scheduled an emergency food enrollment appointment for her. The community organizer offered assistance in enrolling the kids in the summer lunch program. Then I turned my attention to Johnny. I told him about the community garden across the street and told him that if he helped it grow by caring for the plants, then he could take food from it. He didn't need money, only time to help out. The community organizer gave him her phone number and told him the next time she would be working in the garden.

Johnny proceeded to eat the pasta and cheese but threw away all of the vegetables from the pasta salad. I said, "Johnny, why didn't you eat the vegetables. That's the part that comes from the garden, the part that keeps you full, and the part that makes you grow. Most importantly, that's what makes the pasta salad taste good!" He replied that he never ate the vegetables. He never had any at home, and he always throws them away because his friends at school throw them away. He just assumed they were "gross".

"Johnny," I said. "I am going to make you a deal. If I give you another plate of pasta salad and you taste every vegetable, I will let you take the extra bowl I have here home with you."

He perked up and gave me a big smile. "I can do that."

First, he tried a black olive. He said, "Wow! It's salty like fries."

Second, he tried a cherry tomato. "This is what a tomato tastes like? Is this what they use to make pizza sauce?"

"Yes," I replied. "Tomatoes are cooked with other seasoning to make sauce. If you work in the garden, you will learn about the plants that make seasoning."

Then he tried a green pepper and spit it out. "Do I still get the pasta salad even if I don't like [green pepper]?" he asked.

"Yes," I replied. "But please don't throw them away. It took me forever to cut them all up! Push them aside and give them to one of your friends who likes them."

Finally, he tried a cucumber and said, "Umm. . . not as good as a tomato, but I can eat it."

I packed a large department store paper bag with the remaining pasta salad, paper plates, forks, and display vegetables. Johnny eagerly took it and proudly showed it to the rest of his family who had watched his vegetable taste test closely. They congratulated him. Conversation among the kiddos included trying the vegetables that Johnny ate when they got home, total disbelief that I let him keep all the food, and talking about how they were going to work in the garden to make their own food this summer. I was overtaken by how excited they were.

The community service worker and I were laughing as we cleaned up the display and headed back to the office. However, in the car I started to cry a little bit. The kids in the neighborhood were overjoyed with food. Regular, everyday healthy food. They had been offered the healthy food at school and threw it away because they didn't recognize it. How can they be expected to eat well, when they don't know what to eat?

Later that summer, I returned to Summit Lake and ran into Johnny at the "Let's Grow Akron" harvest sale. The same family had been enrolled into a children's entrepreneurship program. The kids were selling vegetables they grew in the garden to earn money for school supplies. I bought four giant zucchinis from Johnny and told him I was going to make zucchini bread with them. He told me that he tasted zucchini bread at Let's Grow Akron and that he loved it. He wanted to make it too.

It took a team of people to change the health outlook for Johnny and his family. The corner store owner was open to changing his business model. The community organizer and I went to a part of town that many people avoid to being this program. And the community service worker stayed and engaged a partner nonprofit to assist in tending the garden and engaging the kids long term. These changes did not cost very much. The recipe for this work included two ingredients: (1) time and (2) trust.

Patients' life experiences may not have given them many privileges that have come easily to care providers. Patients' point of view is often limited by their life experiences, the places they live, and the information sources they have available. Perhaps sometimes the best place for community health education is the neighborhood liquor store.

Why Didn't You Ever Call Me?

Emily George

"Dr. George!" my patient yelled across the sidewalk as we all filed out of our office building as the fire alarm blared in the background. She came hurtling at me, as fast as she could move her 400 pounds of body. "Why didn't you ever call me?" I could see heads turn and stare. Tears were streaming down her face as I focused all of my energy on keeping an even tone and calm voice while secretly wishing I could melt into the crowd and have a security backup. I gently informed her that I did indeed get the encounter from the nurses saying she'd called, but it had only been a couple hours, and I had been seeing other patients that day. I sat her down and we talked about what was going on. She still had a headache, something that had been persistent for some time and started after her last boyfriend had hit her. She was on her way to the emergency room (ER) to get checked out again, and I couldn't convince her otherwise.

Madison (name changed to protect patient privacy) was a 20-something-year-old who frequented the area emergency rooms for various complaints. I became her primary care physician my second year of residency. We got to know each other very quickly. I would receive ER report after ER report, call after call of various complaints. After the first several times I saw her, she came in with a case worker from an area mental health agency. The case worker joined us for the visit with the permission of the patient and interjected quietly but mainly supported the patient with simple verbal and non-verbal encouragers. Madison was every physician's definition of a "difficult" patient. She was a frequent flyer, so to speak, to the point where I finally just scheduled her for an office visit every month to try to keep her out of the ER for complaints that were not emergencies. During her office visits, we would easily address 10 or even 12 complaints, many of which were minor or simply had no physical basis. Her case worker came more and more often, which was a tremendous help.

E. George (✉)
Akron City Hospital, Summa Health System, Akron, OH, USA
e-mail: ebennett@neomed.edu

© The Author(s) 2019
A. Perzynski et al. (eds.), *Health Disparities*,
https://doi.org/10.1007/978-3-030-12771-8_19

She called me after one of Madison's visits to provide some more information that I hadn't been able to elicit. Madison was pretty much on her own. Her family was not involved, and, ultimately, she should have been plugged into the MRDD Board's system, but was tested in school. She lived in an apartment with no oven or stove and didn't have a bed. She slept on the floor. The only thing she was able to "cook" were microwave meals. She had a difficult social life and, in order to find support and love, frequently provided herself for male and female partners. She had significant depression and anxiety that was under moderate control by a local psychiatrist.

Armed with this information, we continued our monthly visits together. She started passing out frequently and the ER visits piled up again. We spent 3 months discussing why she was passing out and what she was feeling before and after. Nothing abnormal showed up on testing. She came to the office one month, and I delved into how she was coping with her current situation. She immediately looked at me, closed her eyes halfway, and slammed back on the exam table. I made sure she was breathing and her heart was beating and checked her sugar and blood pressure, all of which was normal. Her case worker and I started talking to her. As we talked, she would peak open her eyes once in a while, but not respond. After a while, she opened her eyes, sat up, and started interacting. I told her that I thought that her passing out spells were a manifestation of how she was dealing with her current stressors, to which she immediately passed out again. We checked a couple labs and I let her go. The next month, she was in the ER less and less. She went to group therapy more and more. When she came into the office, there was a commotion in the hallway. Our charge nurse came and got me because she had passed out in the hall. I went out to her, talked to her quietly, got her up, and put her in a room. We made sure she was hemodynamically stable and gave her a drink of water. That visit, she was very open to how her stressors were affecting her physical body. She started to understand that when she was anxious or in loud places, she passed out. After that, it stopped. She stabilized. Her case worker helped her get a mattress. She was able to get moved into an apartment with an oven. I felt comfortable enough with her psychiatric stability that I referred her to bariatric surgery for surgical weight loss management.

We continued to have monthly office visits, addressed her many complaints, which, by that point, I could firmly say were psychosomatic, and much of the visit was just reassuring her that everything was fine, she wasn't dying, and she would be back next month to see me. One day she showed up in the clinic hysterical. One of the medical assistants put her in a room and immediately got our behavioral health coordinator (BHC) to see her. The BHC came out of her room wide-eyed. Madison was having an acute psychotic episode. She was suicidal. She was saying she was demon-possessed and that the demons inside of her were trying to get out. Her eyes were blood shot from crying. She was screaming. The BHC said that she was fearful of Madison when she was in the room with her alone because of how aggressive she was talking. She didn't try to hurt anybody, but she was making a ruckus.

Everyone could hear her. I went into her room and completed a medical assessment of her. As I moved to the psychiatric portion of my review of systems, she got agitated. I asked her to expound upon what she had told the BHC. She told me what she had said and then broke down saying that she didn't want to get sent to the ER. She knew the path of what she had said.

As soon as I told her I had to pink slip her for her safety, she freaked. She yelled and screamed and cried. I told her that I would be back with a box of tissues for her and left the room, telling one of the staff to call security because she was going to try to leave. She did indeed try to leave, snarling at anybody who got in her way, but thankfully, the security office is right across the street, and they were in our office within a minute. They caught her trying to go out the office door, guided her back in, all while trying to de-escalate a screaming woman. It took four of them to get her in a room. She tried to grab one of their guns, so she had to be hand-cuffed. I wrote the pink slip and sent her to the ER for psychiatric assessment. While I was completing all the paperwork and calling the psychiatric resident and ER, I could hear from down the hall, "Dr. George, I'm going to find you and kill you," followed and interspersed with a slew of expletives. I checked on her status in the ER throughout the afternoon (she had been my first patient of the day). The psychiatric resident saw her and discharged her straight from the ER. I couldn't believe it. All of that screaming, talk about demon possession, hate, and threats that came from this woman I had taken care of so carefully and diligently for 18 months was just that, screaming, hate, and threats. She wasn't psychotic. She wasn't manic. She wasn't suicidal. She wasn't delusional.

I had a real internal struggle about how to process this information. I felt threatened. She knew where I worked, and I firmly thought she was capable of getting a gun and coming to find me. She didn't have the coping mechanisms to deal with what she viewed as the forceful removal from my office to the ER. I talked to our medical director, a couple of my supervising attending physicians, and our department psychologist. They all encouraged me to dismiss her for her behavior. She put multiple people at risk, and if she came in and saw another provider after acting like that and it happened again, I would feel terrible. The behavioral health specialists in the office helped me the most. They had met with her multiple times and knew her disabilities and viewpoints. They affirmed that if the psychiatrist did not feel that she was psychotic, then she knew what she was doing while she was at the office, and that behavior crossed a line. Even though she had certain disabilities, she still had to be held accountable for her actions.

"Firing" her from my practice was one of the hardest things I did during residency. I was, simultaneously, relieved, exhausted, and disappointed in myself for not being able to be of more help to her. I had spent a year and a half forming a relationship with and doing what I felt was going above and beyond for this person who then threatened me. I did not know, still do not know, how to resolve the turmoil and disparaging feelings I was having.

Part VI
Immigration

Everyone Called Him Crazy

Veronica Cheung

Everyone called him "the crazy guy" – he was known as one of the most difficult patients to take care of by our emergency department (ED). No one could understand him, no one could offer him what he needed, and no one wanted to take care of him. Caregivers would be just as confused and frustrated at him as he was with the health-care system.

This patient was an elderly gentleman who did not speak a word of English. He emigrated here from Vietnam many years ago and still lives alone without a significant other or children. Although he is able to cook for himself, he appears frail. He learned how to use the public transit system, and that is how he travels from his house to the ED.

With close to monthly appearances in the ED for abdominal pain, this Cantonese-speaking patient was a nuisance to everyone. Many times, there were no translators available, and his slurred speech consisting of a mixed dialect of Cantonese and Taishanese made translation even more difficult. He had no primary care provider and had minimal medical records in our electronic medical record system.

I finally got a chance to meet this gentleman after he was admitted to the general medical floors one night for abdominal pain, urinary retention, and lots of yelling and screaming, suggesting to the medical staff in the ED that he must have been in significant discomfort. They allowed the floor team to take care of the rest.

When I first met him, he had hours' worth of stories to tell me. I was relieved that I could understand most of his words and he seemed comfortable. He told me he thought everyone was crazy and that Caucasian people were treating him poorly. He thought they were racist.

From our conversations, I understood that he had abdominal pain and benign prostatic hypertrophy leading to chronic urinary retention. His medications were a disaster; he was not taking the appropriate medications; he was taking them at

V. Cheung, MD (✉)
Case Western Reserve University School of Medicine, Metrohealth Medical Centre,
Cleveland, OH, USA

wrong doses; he did not have any understanding as to what he was being treated for. He also went to multiple pharmacies, so there was not a single pharmacist who could reconcile his medications with me.

After a long talk about his frustrations and his health problems, we were able to direct the right specialists to optimize his care. All his medications were reconciled, labeled with instructions, and explained in Cantonese by me personally. Our team advised discharge to a skilled nursing facility for the interim, given he lived alone and has a Foley catheter in place for his urine retention. He refused the option and made multiple scenes on the floors. The interpreter line could not understand him and I was off work that day. Only after I returned did I find out that he had stored a large sum of cash in his house that he needed to lock up prior to going to the facility. We arranged for a ride to take him home briefly to lock up his money the following day after he reached the facility.

He has been described as a difficult patient, but not to me. I assigned myself as his primary care provider, gave him a few of my cards, and asked him to follow up with me routinely. He thanked me multiple times and was in agreement with our plan, but I have never seen him again in clinic. He never picks up the phone when I call and try to enquire about his missed appointments with me, so I do a routine chart review on him to make sure he is well. It looks like he comes to the ED less often but still has intermittent abdominal pain. I look forward to seeing him again. He has an appointment scheduled with me next week.

Although I imagine that I would never be able to fully understand what it feels to have a communication barrier as long as I live in North America, I can understand what it feels like to be in pain, incorrectly diagnosed, and improperly treated. This patient has taught me the frustrations and less than optimal care for those that have a language barrier in our health-care system. Although we may not be able to always have all interpreter lines available or learn every language in this world, what we can provide is patience.

Headache

Sharefi Saleh

I recently moved from the Middle East to Ohio after the war broke out. It has been a hard transition moving to a new country. I've been blessed, but nonetheless it has been hard. Simple things like going to the grocery store to buy the foods my children and I are used to eating. The foods we like are hard to find. Communication is the hardest. I went to see a doctor a few days ago about my headaches. He was a male Caucasian doctor. He was very polite and receptive. We used a two-telephone system called a language line during our meeting. But how do I explain my situation with someone who is not familiar with the culture or language? Even my simple jokes are lost in translation. How do I explain to him that my husband was killed during a US airstrike on my town? I will never tell him I want to go back home. Who would ever understand how I felt, let alone this doctor? I see the news how they see people from where I come from as just foreign terrorists who are taking over their resources. I was happy living back home before they took away my husband. My children went to a good school and we played at the playground near our home. I was an architect back home – I helped design several of the buildings that have now been destroyed. I will just see him once and get pain meds for my headache. Maybe someday I will be able to go back home; I was happy there – did not have headaches.

S. Saleh (✉)
MetroHealth Medical Center, Cleveland, OH, USA

© The Author(s) 2019

A. Perzynski et al. (eds.), *Health Disparities*,
https://doi.org/10.1007/978-3-030-12771-8_21

Language and Nuance

David Brinkman-Sull

I met James and his wife, Rita (not their real names), when I was a postdoctoral fellow working in a family therapy clinic. They were coming there because it was free to low-income patients and was one of a handful in our community that offered full translation services. They were illegal immigrants from Mexico with two teenage children. James and Rita did not speak any English, but their children were good students and spoke both English and Spanish fluently. We discussed having their daughter translate for them but decided to use an interpreter so that the whole family could be part of the therapy and because family interpreters introduce errors into clinical conversations. James had been cheating on Rita for several years with a younger woman who was part of their community, and when this came to light, it caused scandal for their family in the community.

Some sessions were held with just the couple and some were held with their nuclear family and a few were held with their extended family at their request. Using a translator was a challenge at first and required a shift in the timing of my inquiries and ongoing patience while waiting for responses to be translated. Because therapy relies on the nuance of language at times, I was always left wondering how my words were being communicated and whether their words were being translated accurately back to me. I knew that something was being lost, but it was hard to know how much. We were fortunate to have the same translator for nearly all of our sessions and over time, she became a member of the treatment team and she was treated by the family as an extended family member as well. It took time, but eventually the family came to trust and become comfortable with the interpreter and me, and this opened the door for more frank conversations that were necessary for us to move forward.

D. Brinkman-Sull (✉)
Summa Health System, Case Western Reserve University School of Medicine, Metrohealth Medical Centre, Akron, OH, USA
e-mail: brinkmand@summahealth.org

As day laborers who were in the United States illegally, and as a family with Mexican heritage, they came from and lived in a culture that was foreign to me. Although I assumed they were culturally much more similar to the interpreter, I came to realize over time that they were culturally and ethnically quite different from her as well. I did not think about and was not aware of the concept of health disparities at the time I provided this care. However, I was aware of the importance of being sensitive to cultural differences between therapist and family, and I had tried to make this explicit in the therapy room. To this end, we spent much therapy time discussing the cultural rules and expectations in their community and the morals and values they held and followed. I found that I often made assumptions about their family relationships that were based on my background and culture that were incorrect. They were patient with me and willing to educate me regarding my invalid assumptions. I came to learn that the amount of pressure and anxiety that they felt because of their illegal status in the United States was extreme. The family's immigration status had a daily impact on their family and their daily behaviors and activities. The freedoms and rights that I take for granted as a citizen of our country were not available to this family. I had to frequently adjust my expectations and assumptions about their lives to help me understand their daily reality. The fact that their children were attending local schools and were successful students, who were rapidly increasing participation in American culture, resulted in a challenging discrepancy in the experiences of the two generations living in their household. It also caused their children to at times disrespect and discount the wisdom and knowledge of their parents.

The Case of Baby G

Anirudha Das

At 23-week gestation, an infant was born at the county safety net hospital. The parents were from Nigeria. After landing in the USA as refugees for the first time, the mother quickly developed premature rupture of membranes and preterm labor (likely related to the stress of the travel) and gave birth to the baby (we can call baby G) at just 23 weeks. The mother did not have any prenatal care in Nigeria. The child had three siblings ages 1, 3, and 5 years old. The entire family did not speak any English, and they were from a small ethnic community that spoke a dialect often unavailable via the interpreter line service in the hospital. The Nigerian physician on the hospital staff also needed the interpreter line to communicate with the family.

There were several issues with this child during his 4-month stay in our neonatal intensive care unit (NICU). The child had to get a tracheostomy due to severe bronchopulmonary dysplasia and later a Gastrostomy tube for the inability to take food by mouth. The mother was not able to visit the child regularly due to lack of transportation and money. Baby G had many ongoing and serious health issues including infections and several surgeries.

Tracheostomy care is challenging even for well-prepared families. Nearly half a year had passed when this child was at last stable enough to be discharged home. It quickly became clear that the caregivers were neither interested nor capable of giving proper care of the tracheostomy themselves. This was primarily due to the language barrier. The care team in the hospital tried and failed on multiple occasions to communicate the seriousness of the situation and the necessity for each of the steps involved to keep the baby safe at home.

The child was transferred to a long-term rehabilitation center for further care. Every day was a struggle for Baby G and his family. There is a strong possibility

A. Das (✉)
Cleveland Clinic Lerner College of Medicine Affiliated with Case Western Reserve
University, Cleveland Clinic Foundation, Cleveland, OH, USA
e-mail: DASA@ccf.org

© The Author(s) 2019
A. Perzynski et al. (eds.), *Health Disparities*,
https://doi.org/10.1007/978-3-030-12771-8_23

that this child may never go home with his parents as his needs are far more than the parents can ably fulfill.

In an advanced practice like ours, we have utilized modern technology and therapeutic techniques to help this woman deliver her baby and keep the baby alive. On the other hand, Baby G directs our attention to many areas of disparity where our technologies, therapies and treatments are inadequate.

Lost in Translation

Mircea Olteanu

This is a case of a 58-year-old Caucasian female patient of Greek origin that presented on January 28, 2013, for a periodic dental examination. The patient came with her husband, neither of them fluent in English, both barely able to understand basic English words and almost no medical terms.

After a short discussion, we found out that the patient has a son who speaks English and that he could not come to this appointment because he was working. The patient tried to give me her cell phone saying that she can call him and he will help with translation. I decided to wait to talk to her son until toward the end of the visit so I could discuss treatment needs and options for the patient.

I found out, after checking her Epic chart, that she is a patient in the system since 2004, but she really started to use our services in 2007 when she was diagnosed with diabetes. Her first visit in dental clinic was in May of 2011. She had some dental work done including a lower removable partial denture that she was not wearing due to the discomfort that is caused by it.

After an oral evaluation of the patient, I am ready to discuss her needs and possible treatment plans with her. She calls her son who is available to provide translation over the phone. The discussion went on for about 10 minutes with the phone being passed alternatively between the patient and myself. If the patient needed to ask a question, the son would translate and give the answer back and then repeat it over the phone so the patient hears the answer. I remember it was a difficult interaction and most likely a lot of information was lost in translation and the patient did not leave with a clear understanding of what her needs or options were.

Toward the end of the visit, I tried to adjust the patient's lower partial denture to eliminate sore spots and pressure-creating spots. Because of the discomfort that this process created, the patient did not tolerate it and did not want to continue the process. She asked how much a new partial denture would cost and left without her concern being addressed. Lack of good communication and understanding of the

M. Olteanu (✉)
MetroHealth Medical Center, The Senior Health and Wellness Center, Cleveland, OH, USA

© The Author(s) 2019
A. Perzynski et al. (eds.), *Health Disparities*,
https://doi.org/10.1007/978-3-030-12771-8_24

process and a lack of adjustments in 2011 and 2012 made the end result less than desirable.

Only after the patient left did I have a chance to think about the case and understand how good communication with the patient could have solved many of her concerns. I believe that if I would have approached the first visit concentrating more on her background, understanding her culture, and obtaining just a little bit more information about her medical conditions, I would have been much more successful in getting a positive outcome. I also should have scheduled her for a second visit where her son could be present to discuss her concerns and treatment options.

We encounter similar situations daily as we treat many immigrants. The only variable is the presence of a family member that can translate at the time of the appointment or the degree to which the patient understands English. I had the chance to meet the patient again on February 14 when she came for her dental cleaning appointment. In my attempt to recover from the unsuccessful first appointment, I discussed with her that she should bring her son at the following appointment to discuss one more time what her problems are and what treatment options we have. She seemed interested but a bit concerned that, due to her son's work schedule, she may not be able to make it with him.

Sure enough on February 21 she had to reschedule her appointment for the next week, February 26. At this point I am waiting to meet the patient again and see if we are successful in creating good communication and if the patient's goals are met. I am a little bit reserved as I see that the patient has a bad track record in keeping her appointments: more than 75% cancelled or no-show appointments no matter what medical specialty. A possible explanation for all of those unfulfilled appointments may be the communication barrier, the inability to show up on time for the appointments, or the inability to cancel and reschedule because of the language barrier. I am not entirely sure about the real cause.

The Struggles of the Undocumented

Chris Gillespie

At McCafferty Health Center, we have a large population of immigrants from all over the world. We attract an especially high number of immigrants from Latin America due to the fact that our staff is bilingual in English and Spanish. A 2003 Institute of Medicine study showed that Limited English Proficient (LEP) Americans tend to receive less care, and lower-quality care, than the majority (white) population. For those LEP patients, the hurdles to accessing quality health care can be especially difficult. In addition, if a patient is undocumented, it becomes even more challenging. I would like to describe the experiences of a few of my LEP patients at McCafferty so that we may better understand the hardships they face in life, especially in relation to their health needs.

Patient 1, Male, Age 60

The first patient I would like to tell you about is a 60-year-old gentleman from Guatemala. He came to the United States in 1979 and currently lives alone. He has learned some broken English over the years but primarily communicates in Spanish. He does have an adult daughter who helps him, but she works full time and is frequently unable to come with him to his appointments. He is disabled and unable to work. He is now a US citizen and has Medicare.

The reason for his disability is that he has difficulty walking secondary to nerve damage of his spine from a non-malignant tumor of the spinal cord. The tumor has been resected once previously but has recurred. He does not want to have any further surgeries. He also has diabetes which is not well controlled. Because he spends most of his day sitting he has developed chronic and recurring decubitus ulcers on

C. Gillespie (✉)
Family Medicine, McCafferty Health Center, The MetroHealth System, Cleveland, OH, USA
e-mail: cgillespie1@metrohealth.org

© The Author(s) 2019
A. Perzynski et al. (eds.), *Health Disparities*,
https://doi.org/10.1007/978-3-030-12771-8_25

83

his buttock and sacrum which have led to osteomyelitis (a severe bone infection), several prolonged hospitalizations, and numerous surgeries to repair the wound. Diabetes has contributed to the infections. He also has a neurogenic bladder as a result of his spinal cord tumor which requires him to have a chronic Foley catheter. This makes him susceptible to urinary tract infections.

This patient's medical problems are challenging enough, but he also has the added difficulties of not speaking English well, living alone, walking without a walker, and primarily using a wheelchair. He is a proud man and does not like to ask for assistance. We have tried in the past to get him a home health aide but he has been very resistant and usually refuses. He also faces financial difficulties. He has not been able to work for many years.

Recently he was billed for medical supplies that he never received. He lives in a two-family home and his door is in the back. His supplies were once delivered to the front door. His neighbor never gave him the supplies but he was still billed $274 by our medical supplier. He had to come in to our office and meet with the social worker and financial counselor to address this since he didn't feel comfortable calling the supplier directly with his limited English. Since the supplies were delivered to the correct address he was responsible for the bill. He had to pay it back in monthly installments.

Patient 2, Male, Age 20

The next patient is a young 20-year-old gentleman from Ecuador who arrived in this country only 4 months prior to his first visit with me earlier this year. He speaks only Spanish. He presented to me with multiple physical complaints such as headaches, abdominal pains, nausea, and insomnia. After further evaluation, it appears his symptoms were related to stress.

He came to Cleveland to live with his aunt because his father back home was very abusive toward him, his mother, and his siblings. He has been traumatized by his many violent exposures as a child. He is here now to work and send money back to his mother who is now single since his father abandoned the family.

He is very lonely here and feels very isolated since he has no friends and can't speak English. He was very close to his mother. His aunt is nice to him, but is not very affectionate. We were able to get him connected with our Spanish-speaking behavioral health specialist at McCafferty. He was able to find a job and is doing a little better now but is still very lonely and sad secondary to his traumatic situation.

Kidnapped

Diana M. Kingsbury

The translator and I arrived at a modest home in a neighborhood just outside of downtown. We were halfway through the interview process – at perhaps number 20 or 21 of the 45 we had planned to conduct. The neighborhood and home were much like the others – a bygone reminder of Akron's booming rubber industry days and now representing a new era of the city's history – the resettlement of hundreds of refugees from some of the world's most troubled regions. We approached the home and saw several pairs of shoes lined neatly next to the door. We removed our own shoes and stepped inside.

We were greeted with bows and a quietly spoken "namaste" by the young woman we were there to interview, along with the several family members and neighbors who were also present and who represented multiple generations. They greeted us politely, with smiles, curious about who we were and what we were doing. We greeted them with smiles in return, also curious and aware of the immensity of having to uproot all that you know, leaving behind family, friends, and homes, to live somewhere so far away and different from all you know.

The translator began speaking to the young woman in Nepalese – *We are researchers from a university near here. We are interested in learning more about your experiences of having a baby since you arrived. We would like to know more about who helped you during your pregnancy. This may help us make this experience better for other women. Can we speak somewhere quiet?*

She led us to one of the bedrooms in the home, the beds neatly made, with signs that the room was shared by several people. A box fan whirred from its place in the corner, cutting through the summer heat. The young woman instructed us to sit in two plastic chairs, while she took a seat on the floor, near the fan. She smiled brightly through hot pink lipstick. She was very small, less than 5 feet tall.

D. M. Kingsbury (✉)
Department of Family & Community Medicine, Northeast Ohio Medical University,
Rootstown, OH, USA
e-mail: dkingsbury@neomed.edu

© The Author(s) 2019
A. Perzynski et al. (eds.), *Health Disparities*,
https://doi.org/10.1007/978-3-030-12771-8_26

Her stature and youth, however, were underscored by what seemed like deep knowledge of hardship. We began the interview.

She shared her age, demographic information, her length of time living in the USA, and who she leaned on most for support during her pregnancy. I sat and observed as the translator spoke with her in rapid fire Nepalese. Something was different this time, however, as I noticed a story begin to unfold as the young woman began to speak at length. The translator nodded periodically, asked questions in return, and listened some more. Several minutes had passed as I watched the exchange continue. Finally, the translator turned to me and said "This is what she just shared with me about her experience before coming here" – she asked permission from the young woman to repeat the story to me – and continued.

She told us a story about growing up in Nepal with a mother who lived with an untreated mental illness. She described the challenges of this and the harsh treatment she received from her mother. She had gotten married young and had a baby, but her mother intervened and contacted authorities claiming she was too young. Her marriage ended and the baby was put up for adoption. She married again and this time left Nepal and arrived in the USA with her husband. Her mother, aware that she had left Nepal, contacted authorities in the USA, claiming she had been kidnapped. At the time, she was 17 years of age and was placed in foster care for a year until she was able to return to the home she shared with her husband.

She spoke about these experiences stoically, but brightened into a smile again when spoke about her life now, particularly when discussing the baby she had given birth to the in the USA. This was positioned within the devastation she continued to feel at the adoption of her first born in Nepal. We continued through the interview for an hour, learning more about her life and her pregnancy. She never spoke of regret, fear, or disappointment. She did not refer back to the story she shared with us.

As we concluded the interview and said our goodbyes, I carried the sense of enormity of human experience with me. To understand the depth of the stories another carries with them was a lesson I learned through these interviews I simply wasn't expecting or looking for. I've thought back to this young woman several times since then and am still in awe of her strength and resilience.

Conveying Care

Feras Ghazal

This is a case of a 48-year-old Chinese female who came to the dental department. She was pointing to her lower front teeth. I realized from her facial expressions that she was in pain. This was her first visit to the dental clinic. There was also no information about her dental and medical history. When inquiring the reason for her visit, I noticed that she could barely speak or understand basic English words.

I moved with the patient to the front desk to talk to the interpreter using the telephone since there was no one in the clinic that speaks her language. I asked the phone interpreter to collect information about her chief complaint and the onset, the duration, and the severity of the pain. In addition, I asked via the interpreter a full medical history, current medications, and allergies. After that, I went back with the patient to the clinic dental examination room to complete the exam and take x-rays.

After the oral evaluation, the treatment plan was to pull out her lower front teeth because of the decay and periodontal involvement. We got her up from the dental chair and went back again to the phone system to talk to the interpreter to discuss the patient's needs and possible treatment plan. Explaining the dental procedure to the patient and obtaining the informed consent for extraction were additional steps in the translation process. I had to explain the informed consent to the interpreter first who was unfamiliar with some dental terms. Then, the interpreter translated everything to the patient. Furthermore, post-surgical instruction was another document I had to clarify to the interpreter and made sure that the patient fully understood the consent and the post-surgical instructions prior to signing the consent.

Again, the patient and I went back to the clinic room to start the treatment. Deep inside myself, I had a hidden concern. What would I do if I want to explain something to the patient in the middle of the extraction? Do I need to stop it and go back to the interpreter? Will the patient be able to communicate with the interpreter once I have begun local anesthesia? The extraction went fine with no complications of the procedure. I gave the patient her medications and written post-surgical instructions.

F. Ghazal (✉)
The MetroHealth System, Cleveland, OH, USA

© The Author(s) 2019
A. Perzynski et al. (eds.), *Health Disparities*,
https://doi.org/10.1007/978-3-030-12771-8_27

I asked her to let anyone of her family of relatives who speaks English to explain the instructions again for her because I didn't know how much information she caught from the conversation with the interpreter.

After the patient left, I questioned whether translation over the corded phone translator system was an efficient method of transmitting the information. How can I be sure that all information was delivered to the patient and nothing lost in the middle? Was the quality of care the same to this patient as to an English-speaking patient? Would the patient come back to the clinic where no one speaks her language?

Several months later, I shared this story with my colleague Dr. Olteanu at a group discussion of our health disparities' case narratives. He was shocked by the whole story and asked, "Do you not have the cordless translator phone with headphones in your clinic like we have in mine?" Just 1 week and just US$100 later, we now have a much better translation system solution for my clinic.

Part VII
Disability

I Jump in with Her, Share Her Joy, and Look Out for Her Needs

Amy Zack

New chairs, stone walls, and fresh paint adorn what used to be a discount superstore at the end of a half-vacant shopping strip. The store is now my clinic. A 22-year-old patient arrives as a blast of the fall wind fills the waiting area. She hasn't been seen since the spring and comes with a life full of issues behind her. Her clothes neatly worn, smile bright and clearly feeling well, she checks into the desk for her visit and takes a seat in a chair, much nicer than those she has at home, and under a painting she would never purchase.

Upon her arrival an assistant inquires as to the reason for her visit. The patient states only that she wants to be seen (she thinks she might be pregnant). She is seated in an exam room, texting on her smartphone as she waits.

I notice her name on the schedule and open her arrival status chart. Oh, right, Ms. Jones (pseudonym). I recall her story in its depth, with its many highs and lows. The last time I had seen her she was pregnant; it was unintentional and she decided to terminate the pregnancy. She had been recently released from prison. What was the charge? I was not sure. I knew that she had been incarcerated for a year or more. The first time I saw her was just after a suicide attempt. She had been admitted to inpatient psychiatry and was subsequently discharged on medication with follow-up. In the intervening time she was arrested. At that first visit I had done a full psychiatric history. Twenty or more suicide attempts were what I remembered on that fall day. I vividly remembered her spring visit pregnancy diagnosis, her defiance when stating that pregnancy would not work for her. "I can't even take care of myself, how can I take care of a baby?" I also recalled some relief for her about her decision.

"Hi Ms. Jones, how are you? What can I do for you today?" She looks up from her phone giving me a huge smile that lights up the plain medical exam room.

A. Zack (✉)

Department of Family Medicine, The MetroHealth System, Case Western Reserve University, Cleveland, OH, USA

e-mail: azack@metrohealth.org

© The Author(s) 2019

A. Perzynski et al. (eds.), *Health Disparities*,

https://doi.org/10.1007/978-3-030-12771-8_28

"I'm pregnant, I think," she says. I prepare for her reaction and my heart sinks just a bit, worrying for her that she would feel this was, again, not for her. Yet she seems different. Oh, no, manic maybe? Is she on her meds? Many thoughts were streaming through my mind. I asked her lots of basics. She was unclear how far along she was, though she thought maybe a few months. No meds right now, but doing well, she says. She is living in an apartment, having been released from the halfway house. Two jobs, paying her bills, stable for now. She defensively states she doesn't want medication, the side effects don't work for her, and she wants to do well without them. We talk about screening questions for mania and depression. I think, for now, in this moment, Ms. Jones is stable. I wonder if she can handle this. What will happen later down the road, can I continue her prenatal care here? Is she too high risk? What happens if she again ends up incarcerated, using substances, or worst of all, attempting or achieving suicide? A hundred concerns, a hundred instant judgments all of which indicate my worry that, as a mentally ill patient, she will not be able to handle this.

"Sit up here so I can look at your belly," I state. Again, I have a moment of concealed concern. Ms. Jones, I think you are farther along than a month or two. She has, without question at least a 20-week fundus, late prenatal care, late vitamins, and too late for termination as an option for her. I communicate this to her gently and remind her she still has the option of adoption, hoping she wouldn't feel backed into a corner.

Ms. Jones flashed a beautiful smile and said she wanted to keep the baby and that she felt ready and excited. All of my reservations were swirling around inside, worried for her and for the child. We talked at length about her mental illness. She assured me she was doing well. I think to myself it must be the hormonal changes of pregnancy and worry for after delivery but instead, I refocus. This patient with her long history of mental illness is having this baby and needs all of the help our care team can provide. She communicates her concern about others judging her ability to do this, and I reassure her that the social worker, nutritionist, and the Women Infants and Children program (WIC) will help her do her best throughout the pregnancy. I remind myself that making a judgment about her ability to handle this based on her history would not serve her at all. Instead, I make the decision to jump in with her, share her joy, and look out for her needs, knowing that this will help her feel comfortable seeking the care and assistance she needs now and in the future.

A follow-up visit just 2 weeks later, and the fetus is indeed more than 20 weeks, in fact nearly 30 weeks by ultrasound. And it is a boy. I hold my breath slightly, asking how she is and how she feels about everything. Ms. Jones is working hard, trying to get all the items she needs for the baby. She is proud of her hard work. We again talk about her need to see her psychiatrist, work on a plan, and understand her risk. She has a "high-risk pregnancy" and maybe in other circumstances would have to see an obstetrician who specializes in high-risk pregnancies. I think through the case and decide that she would do better here with a consultation from obstetrics. I resist the guideline that suggested passing of the buck. She is nervous. So am I. The outcome and future lay ahead filled with uncertainty. However, this uncertainty doesn't obviate disaster and failure and does not necessitate this patient relinquish her right to the same care anyone else would have.

It is so easy to read a patient case and a list of problems and medications and make a quick decision about someone, their abilities, their risks, and their future. It is easy to fall into the trap of creating disparity and inequality among risk groups without any intention of doing so. Mental illness certainly colors the lives of those affected by it, but it does not make them any less human.

Rude

Ifeolorunbode Adebambo

I am the attending on a busy inpatient service with a team that is made up of three interns and two senior residents.

A few years ago one of the interns had been taking care of a patient for about 2 days. The intern had been working at the hospital for about 3 months and was gradually assimilating the culture. During his presentation to the team on this day, he seemed compelled to express his frustration regarding his interaction with his patient.

"I'm not sure what is going on but I find this patient very rude and I'm having a difficult time interacting with him." He went on to explain that though he tries to interact with the patient, the patient ignores him and will not look in his direction. He seems not to know who he is or recognize him though he sees him several times a day. He went on to report that the patient would stare at him for minutes without speaking to him and would only talk to him when he, the resident, spoke first.

Usually the other residents would comment and give suggestions, but today there was silence in the room after this was divulged, and all the residents stared directly at me waiting for my comment. Later, I understood they had all had a similar experience.

I looked directly at the intern and said "You do know that the patient is blind." You could have heard a pin drop.

I. Adebambo (✉)
Department of Family Medicine, The MetroHealth System, Cleveland, OH, USA
e-mail: badebambo@metrohealth.org

© The Author(s) 2019
A. Perzynski et al. (eds.), *Health Disparities*,
https://doi.org/10.1007/978-3-030-12771-8_29

Power, Pride, and Policy

Emily George

"Can you fill out short-term disability paperwork for me?" my upbeat, rambunctious, 28-year-old patient asked.

"Of course," I said.

She is one of the most resilient people (not just patients) I know. She was diagnosed with a very rare, debilitating rheumatologic disease and has spent the last several years on steroids, getting infusions, undergoing multiple surgeries—including two tracheostomies—and hospital stays all while working and caring for her two children. This is the first time she ever asked to be on disability. She has always taken pride in working and providing a home and stable living situation for her family. We visited and I filled out her paperwork and got it sent to the insurance company.

A couple of months later, she came back for another visit.

"I don't think I can go back to work," she said.

"Ok," I prompted, "What's going on?"

It turned out that she had worked her way up into a managerial position at a nursing facility and she started to make too much money to qualify for Medicaid. With all of her hospital bills, medical equipment, and medications, she knew she would never be able to afford to pay for insurance, her co-pays, and keep her family safe and healthy. We had a long conversation about her options. Paying for private insurance or even an Affordable Care Act insurance plan purchased on the exchange was out of the question; she just did not have enough resources to be able to afford her medications, which were the things keeping her as well as she was. We discussed not working and going on long-term disability; however, she felt like she wouldn't have any meaning to her life. She was an otherwise well 28-year-old with a challenging disease, but wanted to work and support her family and not live off of the system. The third option we talked about was going back to work at her current

E. George (✉)
Akron City Hospital, Summa Health System, Akron, OH, USA
e-mail: ebennett@neomed.edu

© The Author(s) 2019
A. Perzynski et al. (eds.), *Health Disparities*,
https://doi.org/10.1007/978-3-030-12771-8_30

position, but taking a pay cut so that she would still qualify for Medicaid. She was very disheartened at all three options and felt like she earned her current pay, which I did not doubt. She needed to make a forced choice between working for less or applying for disability.

After multiple discussions with her supervisors at the nursing facility, she was set to return to work with a pay cut. Before that happened she was once again hospitalized and needed a third tracheostomy. For now, her decision is on hold as she is again on short-term disability. I have no doubt we will be having a very similar discussion in the near future and likely throughout much of her young adult life as she struggles with fulfilling what every young adult wants to do, work, but doing so in a financially safe way for her and her family.

What's a Woman to Do?

Mary Jo Roach

I first met Pam when she was 55 years old and moved from her small southern town to the big city. Pam was helping my colleague and I evaluate a bladder management decision aid we had developed for persons with a traumatic spinal cord injury (SCI). While evaluating the decision aid, Pam retold her story about her injury and the many decisions she had to make, or, rather, her clinicians made for her, about how to manage and live with a SCI.

At the age of 29, Pam was a hard-working woman providing for herself and her 13-year-old daughter named Jennifer. Pam worked at the local Piggly Wiggly grocery store for a minimum wage, and Jennifer was going to start high school in the fall. Pam and Jennifer did not have much in terms of luxury but owned a small two-story home that Pam had grown up in. Both had many friends, but Pam's parents had passed and her only sister lived 500 miles away.

On August 25, 1990, Pam was involved in a motor vehicle crash that left her with a C4 traumatic spinal cord injury. As a result, she spent the rest of her life in a wheelchair, she had limited use of her hands, and she did not have any control over her bowel and bladder functions. During acute rehabilitation, Pam concentrated on gaining as much function she could so that she could remain in her home with Jennifer after being discharged.

Rehabilitation went well and Pam gained enough function in one hand so that she could feed herself, but she need assistance with dressing, washing, and all transfers, such as from bed to wheelchair, wheelchair to shower, and wheelchair to car, and for her bowel and bladder routines. Prior to being discharged, Pam's friends banded together and built a ramp for her home, so that she could enter and exit the home, rebuilt the doorways to her bathroom and bedroom so they were wide enough for a wheelchair, and held a fundraiser to buy a portable lift that would assist with

M. J. Roach (✉)
Center for Health Care Policy and Research, School of Medicine, Case Western Reserve University, Cleveland, OH, USA
e-mail: mroach@metrohealth.org

A. Perzynski et al. (eds.), *Health Disparities*,
https://doi.org/10.1007/978-3-030-12771-8_31

transfers from the wheelchair to bed and bed to wheelchair. Pam was extremely grateful to her friends, but there was one big issue that she needed assistance with and that was her intermittent catheterizations (ICs) needed to be done every 3 hours. Her bowel program could be done every week by a home health aide, but her insurance could not pay for an aide to come into her home every 3 hours to perform IC.

Pam's SCI doctor told her that if her daughter could not perform the IC, then Pam would have to go into long-term care and Jennifer would have to be placed with her sister 500 miles away or go into foster care. Pam discussed the options with Jennifer who was adamant that she would do the IC for her mom and so Pam was discharged home. At the age of 12 and into her mid-20s, Jennifer made sure that her school and work schedules were such that she could go home to her mom and perform the ICs. For Jennifer, this meant that she was not able to participate in school sports programs, school clubs, or activities that would have meant staying after school or in the evenings. Also, Jennifer would have to arrange her outings with friends or dating life around her mom's need for her.

As life was getting to a new normal for Pam and Jennifer, Pam met a man and they became romantically involved. Pam decided that since things with Pete were getting serious and she did not want to become pregnant, she had better go back on birth control, so she called for an OB/GYN appointment. She specifically told the receptionist that she was in a wheelchair and asked if that was a problem. The receptionist stated that it would not be a problem. Pam had not been to her OB/GYN since her accident two years prior, so she never expected to encounter the barriers to a pelvic exam or obtaining birth control. Jennifer, now 16, had a day off from school because of parent-teacher conferences and was able to drive her mom to the doctor's office. After parking and transferring her mom into her wheelchair, they came upon the entrance of the building where the OB/GYN office was located; there were two steps to enter. Pam looked around and could not see any ramp or alternate route to take. Jennifer went inside the building to ask if someone could help her lift the wheelchair so that Pam could enter the building. The receptionist and one of the office technicians volunteered to help. The three women were able to lift Pam's chair and get her into the office building.

When Pam was called to follow the nurse into the exam room, the nurse looked perplexed and asked Pam if she could stand on the scale. Pam asked if they had a roll up to the scale because she was tetraplegic and could not stand. The nurse then asked Pam how much she weighed and Pam told her what her weight had been 2 years ago when she had a clinic visit with her SCI physician. The nurse entered that weight into her electronic health record (EHR). Then the nurse left the room and said the doctor would be in shortly. The doctor came in and in a kind voice explained to Pam that the office was not equipped to be able to proceed with a pelvic exam because the office did not have a hydraulic exam table that could descend to a level where Pam could be easily transferred nor did they have a lift where they could get her out of the chair and onto the table. The doctor said she apologized for any inconvenience and that the receptionist did not realize that Pam was in a wheelchair due to a SCI. If she had known this, she would have given Pam another doctor's name who was equipped to handle women with a SCI and in a wheelchair. The doctor gave Pam the name of an OB/GYN whose office was at large urban hospital 150 miles away and the only physician who both would accept Medicaid patients and had the necessary equipment for the pelvic exam. The problem was that Pam would need to hire a wheelchair transport service and the cost of a 300-mile round trip would be over $400, considerably more than she could afford. Medicaid would pay part of the cost, but not the entire cost.

The doctor then asked Pam why she would need birth control given her spinal cord injury. Pam was a bit taken aback but explained that her sexual desire was still intact and that she still got her period, so she assumed she could get pregnant. The doctor took Pam's blood pressure and wrote her a prescription for her birth control pills. Pam was able to get the prescription, but she was not able to have her pelvic exam.

Several years later, Pam has now reached the age of 45. She started to have bleeding between her normal period times, some weight loss, swelling of her legs, and a foul-smelling discharge that she noticed when her catheter was changed. She was not sure if these were normal changes in her body due to her SCI or if it was an indication that something was wrong. So, Pam called her SCI doctor and explained her symptoms. He asked her when her last pelvic exam was and Pam stated that she has not had one since her accident because she could not find an OB/GYN close to her home that had an accessible exam table. The doctor said that she could come to the women's clinic his hospital was associated with and, although far from her home, it was imperative that she have the exam. He had his secretary call the women's clinic and make an appointment for the following day.

The results of the office were not at all what Pam was hoping hear. She was told that she had mid-stage cervical cancer. The doctor was hopeful she could go into remission with treatment if she had the will and support from family and friends that is needed during these times. Pam felt guilty that she did not go for a regular pelvic exam even if it meant coming to a doctor who was 150 miles away. At that time, she just could not have afforded the transportation and her daughter could not take an off from school or, later, risk losing her job to take off work to bring her mom. But, if she had, they may have found the cancer much sooner and the fight to get rid of the cancer might have been less intensive. In the end, Pam was able to fight the cancer and she is in remission. After this experience and other health-care issues, such as a sacral pressure ulcer, Pam moved away from her daughter and her friends in her small town to be closer to the large hospital system where she knows the medical offices and all of the equipment are wheelchair accessible.

Now at 55, Pam tells me that she still revisits her first decision after her injury, having her daughter at 12 years old being the person to provide her IC care and the decision not to go in for a regular pelvic exam. She wished she had been told about all different options for bladder management that were available, but the SCI nurses and doctors only told her about IC and not about the other options, such as, an internal catheter (a Foley). A Foley would have freed her daughter from having to be around every 3–4 hours to do the IC, which would have meant Jennifer could have had a more normal teenage life. The decision to not have her pelvic exams over the years has also meant Pam has had to live with the guilt of cancer and the cancer treatment burden experienced by her daughter and friends.

Adrift in the System

Danielle Massarella

I had the opportunity to see a 17-year-old male who had been referred to the pediatric cardiology clinic after his foster care intake exam resulted with an abnormal EKG. He came to the appointment with a group home staff member who knew none of his past medical history, allergies, or current prescribed medications. He was new to our health system and his electronic medical records were outdated and sparse. The answer to every question I asked this young man to ascertain his cardiovascular risk was "I don't know." He had no family history to share and none of his birth history or even surgical history was known to him.

He was ultimately diagnosed with hypertrophic cardiomyopathy. He was advised against continuing his favorite pastimes, which included basketball and weight training. I had the strong sense that we were lowering the weight of the world onto the shoulders of this young man. Understanding the implications of a diagnosis like this is beyond most 17-year-olds I know; and I felt helpless in the situation as I looked at his "caregiver" across the room, texting disinterestedly on his phone while the attending physician was talking to the patient about our findings. I have not seen the boy since. He was lost to follow-up immediately after this visit. With such a serious condition and scarcely anyone around to care for him, I worry that few things will ever go his way. It just feels like the end of my clinic visit should not be the end of the story or the end of us caring for this young man.

D. Massarella (✉)
MetroHealth Medical Center, Cleveland, OH, USA

© The Author(s) 2019
A. Perzynski et al. (eds.), *Health Disparities*,
https://doi.org/10.1007/978-3-030-12771-8_32

Part VIII
Social Support

Jane in Room 18

Michael D. Paronish

I want to tell you about someone I met; I'll call her Jane. Is there anyone in the audience working in healthcare? Of course…I'm sure you have met her, we all do, all too often. Please forgive me, I am not prepared to answer any questions about Jane. I know where we met, but I do not understand how she found herself here in my care.

Today I was pulled to cover inpatient rounds for a colleague with a resident team in a busy hospital. Nearing the lunch hour already, everyone was happily anticipating having time to eat lunch if we avoided any setbacks. Then the call came…ER Room 18 sepsis due to pneumonia. Upon arrival to the ER, I realize staffing is thin as there have been multiple traumas already today, all requiring activation of many resources for their care. In Room 18, we found Jane.

Jane is an elderly African American woman whom I have never met. She appears older than her chart's stated age. She is visibly ill today, diagnosed with sepsis due to pneumonia. She arrived by EMS and is here alone today. There are no family or friends on their way. Jane is currently not able to engage in verbal communication. I cannot discern if this is due to her current medical illness or related to her schizoaffective disorder. The chart review is not clear about her baseline functioning. She has been here for several hours, but few treatments have been given. Jane did not request treatment; she did not make noise. She suffered in silence, alone, not asleep but not communicating with anyone aside from brief eye movements and eye contact. Without anyone to speak for her, to flag down someone rushing about caring for patients who are more able to communicate their needs, everyone else seemed to not notice Jane in Room 18, alone and quiet.

I requested that the already ordered, but not yet initiated, treatments including IV fluids and antibiotics be started immediately. I know that Jane's outcome worsens with each hour delay in fluid resuscitation and appropriate antibiotic therapy. I then find myself justifying the inconvenience while explaining the importance of deliver-

M. D. Paronish (✉)
Family Medicine, Mercy Health, Boardman, OH, USA

© The Author(s) 2019
A. Perzynski et al. (eds.), *Health Disparities*,
https://doi.org/10.1007/978-3-030-12771-8_33

ing this care here in the busy emergency setting for Jane rather than transferring to the floor and waiting for the admission processes and protocols to be fulfilled, followed by the pharmacy to verify the medicines, all of which would likely delay treatment by several additional hours. Ultimately Jane received the treatments prior to transfer. I finished rounds today by explaining to my team of trainees including residents and medical students that they must each advocate for the best care possible of all of their patients. My lesson today: sometimes a patient like Jane who does not request treatment or make any noise at all can actually be quite ill and in need of their help. There should be no cracks to slip through.

I filed a safety report to notify administration of my perception of our systems' shortcomings treating Jane today. I cannot help but wonder what allowed me to encounter this situation. Will it ever be fixed? Did Jane's inability to request help contribute? Did her lack of family or friends to advocate on her behalf place her in jeopardy? Was it Jane's mental illness? Surely in today's work environment it cannot be her race, right? Did the multiple traumas with the constant overhead pages droning on "Trauma ETA 5 minutes" really require all the attention they received? What would have happened if Jane's arrival had been paged overhead? Will my teaching point be remembered? Will I have the energy to continue to work to overcome disparities when I notice? How many patients like Jane in Room 18 have I not noticed? Will these future doctors have the confidence to speak for Jane when they meet her?

Am I a Strong Person?

David Sperling

My family and friends (and even my doctor!) think I'm a strong person, but I don't see it that way. I just do what I need to do to get through each day. Taking care of my family, friends, and sometimes even complete strangers is actually what keeps me going.

Sure, between my diabetes, heart problems, stroke, back pain, and depression, I have had my own health challenges. None of those problems has knocked me to the mat, though. Everyone has challenges; these are mine. Most days, I just take my meds and watch my diet as best I can.

My doctor tells me I have to stay active. No problem there! My son broke up with his girlfriend and I get to take care of their boy, my 2-year-old grandson, James. I must confess that the days I watch him I truly understand why God designed us to have babies when we are young! He is a bundle of energy and keeps me running. I'm exhausted at the end of my days with him, but those are the best days of the week.

The days I don't have James, I enjoy myself preparing and serving dinner to 100+ hungry souls at my church. It breaks my heart to see some of our repeat "customers," especially the young moms and their kids. I'm so blessed to be able to give back this way.

My husband was just diagnosed with throat cancer, so we are running back and forth to a bunch of different doctors, trying to get a straight answer about his treatments. He also has his share of health issues including back pain and has been addicted to pain meds, so I have to lock up my pain meds so he is not tempted to dip into my stash. It is hard having to lock up my meds so my own husband is not tempted to use again, but we both understand this is for the best.

D. Sperling (✉)
Department of Family and Community Medicine, Northeast Ohio Medical University, Rootstown, OH, USA
e-mail: dsperling@neomed.edu

A. Perzynski et al. (eds.), *Health Disparities*,
https://doi.org/10.1007/978-3-030-12771-8_34

Am I a strong person? I don't know. I don't even think about that. I just do what I need to do. Honestly, I think I get at least as much back as I give. My faith, family, and friends keep me going. I think I'd be bored and feel useless any other way (although, I confess, I would be willing to give it a try sometimes!).

Part IX
Addiction and Substance Use

You Can Give Me Something

Imola Osapay

A 50-year-old bald, elderly looking, white male with a gray-white unkempt beard, worn light jeans, and a white button-down shirt was sitting nonchalantly in the examination room when I walked in. He was new to our practice and he had an agenda. I could not take a breath or ask a question as he started with his story. He was in a motor vehicle accident 20 years ago, had undergone back surgery, and was now in pain management, being treated with chronic opiates. He had been on fentanyl patches and hydromorphone; recently, his pain management physician had decreased his doses. He wanted opiates from me. As he told his story he stood up and was hovering over me; I was eyeing the door; and I was feeling threatened.

"Our policy is no controlled substance prescriptions on the first visit," I told him, hoping that would be the end of it.

"Come on doc, you know and I know you can give me SOMETHING," he said.

I was still a resident at that time and used the excuse of, "Ok, let me ask my supervisor," knowing well that I was just buying myself time to take a deep breath and go back with a "No."

He was the first patient that day and he held me in the room for more than 30 minutes. I already had other patients waiting. When I went back to tell him that our policy is our policy, he was already upset.

He was cursing, "This is bullshit," and marched out and slammed the door.

I was relieved, thinking hopefully he will not be back.

A year and a half later, I saw his name on my schedule. I knew where this was going to go so I used the Ohio Automated Rx Reporting System to check on his record of prescription opiate use even before I went in the room. He again was wearing a white button-down shirt and light jeans and looked like he was even much older than before. I found out that he had gone through rehabilitation last year.

I. Osapay (✉)
Barberton Area Family Practice Residency Program, Summa Health System,
Barberton, OH, USA
e-mail: iosapay@summahealth.org

© The Author(s) 2019
A. Perzynski et al. (eds.), *Health Disparities*,
https://doi.org/10.1007/978-3-030-12771-8_35

Shortly after he got out of rehab, his youngest son committed suicide. He had used any and all street drugs he could get his hands on in the previous year including IV heroin. He wanted to stay clean, maybe pick up writing again as he was a writer, and pick up his relationship with his other two sons and his grandkids.

He had been married, but his wife died a long time ago, and he had not had anyone else significant in his life. He was a published writer, but had no more motivation to write, and just did not know what to do with all his time now, off drugs. He wanted something to help with his pain and he said he had nausea and maybe I could get him some Phenergan. I was agreeable and suggested NSAIDs and increasing the gabapentin he was already prescribed, and I sent him down to get basic lab testing done as well as Hepatitis-C (HCV) and HIV tests.

The HCV and HIV tests were positive, so I called him to make a close follow-up appointment and inform him of the results. He wanted to keep this information confidential; he would not be telling his children to burden them. He also informed me he was feeling down, wanting to use again because it was the 1-year anniversary of his son's suicide. To my surprise when I suggested seeing a counselor/therapist he was agreeable so I quickly got him the numbers to call and address to go to. I was starting to feel that maybe he was going to turn around, and then he asked me for more Phenergan. I knew it was inappropriate, but I felt this might be what kept him responsive to my suggestions about his care.

The next time I saw him he had seen the infectious disease specialist who was "running more tests" but had not seen the therapist.

"What could they do anyway?" he asked. After that he disappeared, did not follow up with me, his viral testing, or with infectious disease.

Stalemate

Brian Bachelder

My next patient to be seen during office hours is the typical one whose name is instantly recognizable and causes a shiver much like what a sour candy ball does to your mouth. The interaction is pleasurable enough, but the end result is always disagreeable.

He is an elderly black male who always has a smile and a friendly handshake but still seems frail. As you discuss his health issues you notice the leathered, tattooed skin and the disheveled appearance of his clothes. Then after a few minutes, he begins his usual rocking motion in the chair, a compensatory action that I attribute to his history.

Despite his age and against the odds, he is a crack addict that lives with 10+ other men in a crack house. He smokes cigarettes despite a history of chronic obstructive pulmonary disease (COPD). He panhandles to supplement his social security benefits, and the office staff all know him from "his corner street office." He claims to have quit both cigarettes and crack several times but has always fallen back to the addiction of both. He frequently misses office appointments, even for follow-ups after ICU stays on a ventilator. He skips his antihypertensive medications regularly and his blood pressure is frequently uncontrolled. He refuses flu and pneumonia vaccines because of possible "bad effects." Social service consults have been ineffective as well.

I think of his slowly failing health and my own poor health maintenance scores from his care. Should I continue to flail away at his social situation and habits that I know will not change, or should I try to develop a new paradigm where I only manage his decline with the acceptance of the fact that he will continue to overutilize the health-care system?

So I enter the room and he greets me with a brief smile. After several years of working together, he has learned to trust me. He knows that I will not force my

B. Bachelder (✉)
NEOMED, Rootstown, OH, USA
e-mail: bbachelder@centerstreetclinic.org

advice upon him, and I have learned how much he will accept. I refill his COPD and blood pressure meds, and we discuss his crack use and smoking. I express my concern for him, and he promises to do better. The usual. I sigh—no new problems but no progress. Stalemate.

Trapped

Richard Berry

I turned 54 this year. I live in Cleveland, I was raised in a modest neighborhood and am part of a family that could provide but we're nowhere near wealthy. My schools were not great. I was lucky enough not to have the same drug- and gang-associated violence as some of the places my friends lived in. Seeing a doctor was never a consideration as healthcare on a low salary just wasn't an option. That was for rich people.

I graduated high school and never had felt like college was for me, something, I later wondered if it would have changed things for me. I worked several jobs, mainly in services like customer care and waitressing, and at that time I thought I was doing well. I had a roof over my head, I had money, and what I thought was a stable relationship.

It was these days of disposable income that the alcohol started; initially it was at weekends, weekends feel good, and then I also wanted to have "good" midweeks too. I never realized, or believed that alcohol could ever be a problem. I could drink when I wanted, I could stop when I wanted and there were no health issues as a result of alcohol. No health insurance and no symptoms to me meant healthy.

I'm not sure at the time if the alcohol led me toward bar work or the bar work led to the increased drinking—by this time the drinking was a priority and made time-lines a little hazy. I started to convince myself that I *had* to drink, how on earth could I work full time in a bar and not drink, "just to be sociable you know."

The same salary that was great for a single woman suddenly didn't seem as prosperous for somebody who wants that nicer house and wants to provide that little more for her family. Alcohol was no longer a social tool but had in fact become a coping tool. How could I ever get a better job while never being sober enough to drive to an interview and having an overwhelming anxiety and depression when sober enough to function?

R. Berry (✉)
Department of Family Medicine, The MetroHealth System, Cleveland, OH, USA
e-mail: rberry@metrohealth.org

© The Author(s) 2019
A. Perzynski et al. (eds.), *Health Disparities*,
https://doi.org/10.1007/978-3-030-12771-8_37

Somehow during these 3 years of never going 3 days without a drink I ended up owning the bar that I worked in. I convinced myself that this was a great idea and a positive move for myself. Business ownership comes with the ability to define your own destiny, make your own (and more) money and gives a sense of ownership over something. I was not going to need to drink to cope and had the bonus of living on-site to free up some disposable income.

The vision faded after poor business brought about more drinking, financial concerns led to more drinking, a failed relationship, more drinking, and an apparently trustworthy manager led to more drinking. This was the time I accepted my future and realized that I did need alcohol more than it needed me. If care had been an option at this time, I may have been persuaded to quit had I been educated about what could happen.

Several years passed in a drunken blur before the health issues started, the ones that I convinced myself could have happened to anybody. Subsequent relationships including my current one seemed to be based on one common denominator—alcohol. This brought double the problems.

Everything changed the day I had the chest pain and the breathing problems. That day, the last thing I remember is the emergency medical team and how I told, them how I was fine, how I am running a business that cannot cope without me, and how... I don't really remember any more than that.

The tube was still in my throat when I woke up. The other tubes were still in my arms. My first thought was wondering how long I would be here until I could get back for a drink. I really wanted a drink. After the tube was removed I was told about the cardiac arrest, the failing kidneys, and the failing liver. I was told I was lucky to be alive. That is a very subjective statement to make.

That night I started to blame alcohol for my problems like it was a person with feelings and intentions. *It* did this to me, *it* damaged my heart, *it* damaged my liver, I did none of this, *it* knew what *it* was doing all along. As days went past the realization set in. I still saw alcohol as a living thing but at least started to understand that it was my choice to beat it or my choice to roll over and die. I bargained with myself at first—get through a week and you can have *one* beer, cut down 5 days a week but celebrate at weekends. The stupidity of my thoughts luckily set in before I was well enough to be discharged. It had to be all or nothing, and with newfound motivation, it would be the easiest thing I had ever done. As my heart, liver, and kidneys grew stronger, I thought I had got away with this very close encounter with death.

That was when the real problems started. The constant craving, the constant pain in both feet. I felt trapped in a job where alcohol still talks to me on a daily basis. I am still not aware if these problems existed before the hospital or started after, did the alcohol hide these problems? Every time I saw the liquor bottles I wondered if they could hide these issues again, how easy would it be to find out. The Gabapentin and the Lyrica doesn't take it away and the Oxy I get off the street when I can afford it only gives hours of relief.

So far it has been 6 months without regular alcohol—I did have a beer when I moved to a new house which is ironic as it was a move I made to get away from the alcohol. Alcohol still talks to me on a daily basis, and I am sure it always will. I am clear headed, the business is doing well without me, and there is once again some purpose. I will forever be an alcoholic that doesn't drink as I am not strong enough to ever be a true ex-alcoholic.

Part X
Aging

Growing Old in a New World

Tamer Hassan Said and Hardeep Gill

Case 1

A 77-year-old male patient from Puerto Rico with past medical history of COPD, hypertension, type 2 diabetes, coronary artery disease with history of coronary artery bypass graft, atrial fibrillation, and chronic kidney disease stage 4 was admitted with right upper quadrant pain and jaundice. Initial evaluation did show extrahepatic biliary obstruction due to pancreatic mass suspicious for malignancy. Patient had percutaneous transhepatic drain which was complicated by sepsis due to acute cholangitis. Once stabilized he was transferred to a skilled nursing facility. His renal function continued to get worse. Given Futile Prognosis, Multiple Discussions were conducted with Patient and Family Regarding Goals of care using the Interpretor line: particularly in terms of pursuing pancreatic biopsy and possibly dialysis in near future.

The patient initially elected to pursue all treatment modalities.

Later on, a family friend expressed concerns that this patient was not understanding everything over the phone and family members lacked the understanding of the complexity and seriousness of these diseases. We elected to use a live interpreter for the patient. His cognition was further assessed, and the severity and nature of the disease were rediscussed.

T. H. Said (✉)
University Hospitals Cleveland Ohio, Case Western Reserve University, Cleveland, OH, USA
e-mail: Tamer.Said@UHhospitals.org

H. Gill
Houston Methodist Primary Care Group, Houston, TX, USA

© The Author(s) 2019
A. Perzynski et al. (eds.), *Health Disparities*,
https://doi.org/10.1007/978-3-030-12771-8_38

Case 2

A 66-year-old Serbian patient with prior medical history of hypertension, uncontrolled diabetes mellitus with hemoglobin A1C of 10.4, was seen for a follow-up for diabetic foot ulcer. The language line was used in the clinic during all clinic visits. She had four visits to the clinic with blood sugar recordings in the 300 range. Her foot ulcer was 12×2 cm with poor healing. During her next follow-up appointment, the patient was interviewed with the assistance of the Serbian-speaking interpreter. She was given Was given instruction both verbally and written in the Serbian language. Her hemoglobin A1C trended down to 7.8 on her next test. She had improved healing of her ulcer.

Case 3

A 72-year-old Indian female with history of asthma, hypertension, and hyperlipidemia was seen in clinic for a follow up visit. She consistently had blood pressure readings over 180 despite continuously adding and increasing her doses of antihypertensives. She was accompanied by her son who interpreted for her. She was seen by a physician who spoke Hindi and was familiar with her cultural background. It was discovered that she only took her medications on days she did not feel good so that her medication could last longer. She was explained the rationale of taking her blood pressure medications daily in a culturally recognized fashion. Dietary education was provided based on her dietary habits. Follow-up appointments at 3 and 6 months showed a great improvement in blood pressure recordings; her blood pressure was 154/76 and 140/80, respectively.

Part XI
Technology

Problems with My Computer: The Electronic Path Not Taken

David J. Mansour

Mrs. MZ comes in for a routine follow-up visit. She has long-standing diabetes, hypertension, high cholesterol, obesity, and generalized arthritis. She has mild non-proliferative diabetic retinopathy with mild dry macular degeneration; her vision is poor. She reports feeling okay with current medical therapy. She initially begins the visit with frustration about how difficult it was to get an appointment with me. In many years of seeing her, MZ has never missed an appointment and is usually seen every 3–4 months regularly. MZ complains that she repeatedly sent emails to get an appointment, to me directly, and finally tried to contact the office directly by phone. I review her chart as I cannot remember her emails to me directly. I do not see any patient emails in our medical record. I further review today's appointment scheduling. It appears that MZ made the appointment in person as I do find a nurse triage note from 1 week ago in which one of our primary care nurses discussed her needs and provided a follow-up visit. I asked her about her troubles with the phone as I have heard that sometimes our phone system leaves patients frustrated. MZ says that she called at least three times and waited on line for 10–20 minutes. She became increasingly upset at the electronic phone system. She felt that she could not understand the electronic voice and further missed opportunities to key in the correct number for speaking directly to a person. She felt frustrated that she could not hear the options well enough and had trouble pushing the correct button on her cell phone and home phone quickly enough. She finally gave up and decided to walk in to see me. MZ was seen by the nurse as she became agitated while trying to use the self-check-in kiosk. The patient service representative ushered MZ up to the second floor primary care office for help in scheduling after noticing her frustration when trying to use the automated check-in kiosk.

D. J. Mansour (✉)
CWRU School of Medicine, MetroHealth Internal Medicine – Pediatrics,
Cleveland, OH, USA
e-mail: dmansour@metrohealth.org

During our review of her medications, MZ brings up a concern over not having sufficient medication refills. She feels that she does not have any refills left. We review the screen with her current medication list. The dates of refills and renewals stored in our electronic medical record (EMR) are markedly different than what she remembers. Additionally, she has talked with the pharmacist reading directly from a near empty refill bottle and was informed that there were no more refills left on that prescription. We agree to refill these medications. Upon further discussion with the pharmacist, it is apparent that MZ has several different prescriptions at the pharmacy. It is true that the specific prescription with number 211 for hydrochlorothiazide has no refills left. However, MZ currently has two other back-to-back hydrochlorothiazide prescriptions of 90 days each with three refills. The pharmacist concludes that the pharmacy tech did not review all of the outstanding prescriptions. This is common for patients who use the automated refill line as well as the lack of review of all prescriptions by busy pharmacy technicians. The patient is informed of this and expresses frustration about this situation. She asks that she receive paper prescriptions from now on and will keep them in her possession until the refills are needed.

Later during the next week, MZ calls repeatedly and shows her frustration with our primary care nurses about the lack of responses to her emails and the absence of feedback on her normal hemoglobin A1C value of 6.6. She exclaims that she has wanted to know the results and asks if I am on vacation in that there has been no response and no letter in the mail. I have taken the time to personally call her as the nurse feels upset from being scolded. During the course of the telephone interview, it is clear that MZ has not been checking her e-mails nor receiving the results of her latest blood work. A review reveals that I have released the results via the patient portal and have attached a short explanation of the results. MZ becomes increasingly upset when questioned about the exact steps that she used to attempt viewing the results in the patient portal. She exclaims, "Do you think I am dumb or something? The computer does not work. This makes me want to find a new physician." I attempt to reassure MZ that we can provide care without requiring her to use the patient portal. She suggests that she will consider it. I do not hear from MZ for 3 months and later get word that she has transferred her care from our clinic to a different, nearby small local practice after 10 years as my patient. Her daughter whom I still see feels that she is happier and seems content in a "low-tech" practice.

Lost Without a Map

Adam Perzynski

As it occasionally happens, I was running late. I was due to present findings of my recent research on the digital divide at *Net Inclusion '18*. The research findings were exciting; based on an analysis of nearly 300,000 patients, we determined that a government-sponsored free public Wi-Fi system had increased health-care access and improved communication between patients and their doctors. I was thrilled to be able to present the work at a large session that would include everyone in attendance at the meeting, several hundred researchers, and other leaders. Somehow my enthusiasm did not prevent me from being late. I was travelling from a small project meeting in Cleveland's University Circle to the conference which was about 4 miles away at the Global Center for Health Innovation. I had allowed just enough time to park and walk and catch my breath before taking to the podium.

After parking in the garage beneath Cleveland City Hall, I began a brisk walk to the Global Center. I decided that the mild weather was just nice enough to walk outside. Chest heaving and within about 100 feet of the Global Center, I heard a quiet question, but couldn't make out what was said, and to be honest, I was so focused on the door I did not even see who was speaking.

The voice said again, slightly louder, "Is this 15[inaudible] St. Clair?"

"I'm not sure. I don't think so." I managed to huff out between breaths.

I looked at the man. He was about my age, dressed in a winter coat and pajama pants, carrying a black plastic garbage bag over his shoulder in one hand, and he held a small blue slip of paper in his other hand. He was strong, unshaven, and clearly lost. He was black, tall, and somewhat thin of stature but had muscular hands.

A. Perzynski (✉)
Center for Health Care Research and Policy, The MetroHealth System,
Case Western Reserve University, Cleveland, OH, USA
e-mail: Adam.Perzynski@case.edu

© The Author(s) 2019
A. Perzynski et al. (eds.), *Health Disparities*,
https://doi.org/10.1007/978-3-030-12771-8_40

My first thought to myself was regrettable, "Oh for heaven's sake this better not take long my session is starting any minute and if I am late that will be a total embarrassment." My face was now surely reddened, and I had broken into a light sweat from the brisk walk.

"No. For sure this is not St. Clair. We are actually standing nearer to Lakeside. St. Clair is over there. In fact, that building right there is #1 St. Clair. What is the address again? Where is it you are going?" I asked these questions with all the patience I could muster while thinking to myself that there has to be a rapid solution to this problem, but what kind of person am I if I do not help this man who seems so much like me, just trying to get where he needs to go?

The man seemed a little confused by my questions and replied, "I have an appointment." He then offered to show me the blue slip of paper.

"Oh, Care Alliance, 1530 St. Clair. I don't know which direction that is, but I definitely know Care Alliance." There were three locations on the blue slip, but a checkbox was checked next to the St. Clair location. There was also a time indicated, 11:15 AM. This is the same time I was due to give my talk. I looked at my wristwatch, and it was 11:00 AM. It seemed like we might be a long way from 1530 St. Clair given the size of that number, relative to #1, which was the building 100 feet away.

Care Alliance is a non-profit community health organization. They are primarily known for their nearly 30 years of work in providing health-care and other services to the homeless population of Cleveland. They have a group of outreach workers who visit places in the city where homeless individuals can be found, and they help to connect them with medical appointments and other services.

This man might have already walked a long way today. Then I thought of something, "I've got this." I thought to myself proudly. I reached into my right-front pocket and pulled out a newish, fast, and sleek smartphone.

"What is the address again?" I asked.

"1530 St. Clair."

"Alright, and we are pretty much at #1 St. Clair."

Tap, tap, tap, and a microsecond later, I have directions and a map to Care Alliance.

ETA 6 minutes.

Wait, no that's not right, that is by car.

Tap, tap.

"It's twelve minutes that way." I point east.

"On the right hand side of the street. About 5 blocks."

"Good luck to you, I'm sorry I have to run and give a talk in there." I point at the Global Center.

The man said his name, and I have now forgotten it. I won't pretend here and use a pseudonym. We shook hands. I walked 100 ft. east, not looking back as I was now sure that the session organizer was beginning to get concerned about my absence.

"You coming?" My phone buzzed with a text message.

"Right outside." I texted back.

A man in a gray suit holding his phone with headphones in walked up to me as I was entering the building. "Thanks, I'm from out of town, I didn't know what to say or do. I don't really know my way around here myself and had to ask directions to find this place."

"I'm just glad I thought of a way to help." I said.

To this day I am in disbelief that these events happened. However, nothing that happened on that day was a coincidence. I spend my time doing research on the digital divide and health care because many people do not have Internet access, Internet-enabled devices, and/or the skills to use them. The digital divide is actually creating new health disparities. Those of us with smartphones and data plans have advantages in accessing and using health services that others simply do not. Things are as bad here in Cleveland as they are anywhere in the United States. It took me just a handful of seconds to find directions to a health clinic. This young man did not have a smartphone. Standing there on the podium, I could not help but think that my scientific presentations, my published articles, and this narrative have not changed anything. Yet.

Part XII
Education

Health>Education>Health

I first met Carmendita as she was graduating from high school and needed her physical to go to college. Carmen, a bright, African American female, was so excited to be going to Muskingum University. The first person in her family to go to college, she had a full academic scholarship and planned to become a veterinarian. She had younger siblings and wanted to show them that with hard work, they could go on to higher education, too. As a first-generation college attender and oldest of four myself, I spoke with her about the challenges and future rewards. Carmen grew up in the inner city of a declining rust belt city and was interested in helping her family financially as well. She looked forward to being able to help younger siblings and her mother when she was able to become a vet.

Carmen did well in her first year of college, in pre-professional classes. There were challenges, but nothing that she could not handle. She completed her first year, made some money over the summer in her summer job, and went back to Muskingum for her second year.

When she came home for Christmas break, she made an appointment to see me. She noted some pain in her fingers and a little discoloration on the tip of her left index finger. At the visit, the fingers were not swollen, and the small circular area was not concerning, and she thought she might have pinched it. I said we would watch it and see her back at spring break. But just in case it was Raynaud's, I started her on a calcium channel blocker.

As it often happens in clinics with medical residency programs, she was seen by resident physicians for a few visits, and when I next saw her, her fingers looked like sausages, and there appeared to be auto-amputation at the tips of several fingers. Suspecting a rheumatologic disorder, I tried to refer her to a rheumatologist.

J. M. Spalding (✉)
Department of Family and Community Medicine, Northeast Ohio Medical University,
Rootstown, OH, USA
e-mail: jmspaldi@neomed.edu

© The Author(s) 2019
A. Perzynski et al. (eds.), *Health Disparities*,
https://doi.org/10.1007/978-3-030-12771-8_41

She had no insurance at that time and no money for the upfront payment expected by the rheumatologist. This was before the Affordable Care Act and her only choice was self-pay.

She had to drop out of college due to the pain and inability to use her fingers. I was able to get a rheumatologic consult by phone and started her on medication. Because of her financial concerns, we treated her with steroids to try and control her symptoms. Unfortunately, the symptoms worsened, and she developed pericarditis, requiring hospitalization and a pericardial window. We were able to get a rheumatology consult at this time but were only able to get recommendations for a tapering dose of steroids and no ability for long-term follow-up with rheumatology.

Now Carmen had a chronic debilitating disease, large hospital debt, inability to hold a job, and no prospects for insurance. Our next recourse was to try and get disability coverage for a seemingly healthy (the only thing you noticed if you looked at her were the gloves that she wore constantly) 20-year-old young woman. Several attempts to obtain disability lead to several denials. She was not able to get disability which would allow her to get Medicaid and to get the insurance that she needed.

And this is where I left her. Young, disabled, without insurance. I moved to another town, losing touch with her and her doctors. I often wonder about how her and how she is faring in this medical environment. Did she get the help she needed? Was someone able to intervene? Did she ever return to school? How did her family deal with her illness? And how am I dealing with her illness, knowing that I left her without seeing the problem through?

Working with Carmendita made me aware of health disparities in this country. I wish I could say that I was able to effect change in the system but I can't. I can say that I think of Carmendita often when I hear students and residents talk about non-compliant patients. I remind them of social disparities and that patients are not willfully noncompliant but socially nonadherent for a number of reasons. Our job is to look for the reasons for nonadherence and help the patient to overcome those obstacles to health. Carmendita's story lives on through these interactions, inspiring future physicians.

I Don't Know Why I Brought the Bottle

Joseph Daprano

This narrative was written by the physician in the manner of speech used by the patient. The patient approved this story for publication after listening to it being read to him by a nurse when the physician was not present. The patient remarked "This is the life God gave me and I want to share it in any way I can."

My name is WB. I grew up in the deep south in the 1950s. Jim Crow told me what to do. I was born into a family of eight. My brothers and sisters were older. I didn't go to school. When I was old enough to start school, all my brothers and sisters were already working in the fields. There was no one to walk me to school. Momma didn't want me to walk alone when I was that small. I wanted to go to school. I wanted to go badly. And I got my chance. When I was bigger, I walked alone. That was hard. But my teacher was harder. Why did he expect me to know all this stuff? I started late. He hit me on the head when I gave a wrong answer. So I gave no answers. I came late. Then I stopped going. I went to the fields. No, I never learned in school. I never learned to read. I never learned to write. I did learn my numbers. I had to count the bales. I learned how to drive. I left the south my first chance. Drove right up to Cleveland. I got a job as a truck driver delivering meat. I started as the driver and I had a helper. I could lift those half cows. I could throw those boxes of meat in the truck. I learned the streets real good. I couldn't tell you the names from the signs but my helper told me the names. I learned the names of all the people and places we delivered and how to get there from him. And I could count the money. I was always real careful to count it good. I drove all over Cleveland delivering the meat. My boss knew he could depend on me. I worked for that company for 20 years. I had a family. I made sure they all went to school.

Nobody knew I couldn't read. Not my boss. Not my kids. I knew. I tried to learn through one of those programs. It didn't work. I figured, if I made it this long not knowing how, I should be fine. But then I had headaches and the doc told me my blood was high. He told me I had to take medicine to lower it. I didn't know why. I didn't ask. I didn't like what the medicine did to me so I didn't take it. I went to that

J. Daprano (✉)
The MetroHealth System, Case Western Reserve University School of Medicine, Cleveland, OH, USA
e-mail: jdaprano@metrohealth.org

doctor for a year. Every time I went he said my blood was still high and I needed more medicine. He kept giving me more medicine and sometimes I took it. Sometimes I didn't. I wanted a new doctor.

I found a new doctor. I saw the new doctor for a while. He told me the pressure in me was like the pressure in a tire. If it went too high in a tire I knew what happened. He said if my blood went too high it could explode in my brain and give me a stroke. I know what that is. I have friends who can't walk because of that. I took my medicine. My pressure was still too high. My doc asked me one day to bring in my medicine bottle. I forgot to for a long time. When I came in that day with it I knew what was going to happen. I walked up to the lady at the desk. She handed me a paper I couldn't read. She always handed me this from the first time I came to see this doctor. I always took it. I never told her I couldn't read. Then she told me to drop it in the slot in the door. I always did that. Then the nurse called me back and asked me a bunch of questions. Just like before, she never asked me if I could read. Just if anyone was hurting me or if I had any falls. She took the paper from me and wrote some things on it and told me to go back to the lobby. She never asked me if someone helped me understand what my doctor wants me to do. I would have told her about how my girlfriend reads to me. She helps me with all that stuff.

I had my medicine bottle. My doc called my name and I went into his office. I liked this guy. I don't know why. He didn't grow up having Jim Crow tell him what to do. I doubt he ever worked in the fields. He knew how to read. He was white. I am not. He asked me to show him my medicine. I did. He asked me, like he always does, when did I take my medicine. I told him sometimes in the morning and sometimes at lunch. He asked me to read my bottle so I told him no. He said how do you feel about your reading. I told him. I told him I couldn't read.

I hadn't ever told anyone that. I don't know how I felt. He asked why I hadn't told him before. I said because I wasn't sure I wanted to tell. He said, I guess I didn't ask. I told him why I couldn't read. He took the pills out of my bottles and we looked at each one and he told me what each one was and when to take it. I started taking my medicines the way he said would help me not get a stroke. I don't know why I brought the bottle that day. I could have just gone to a new doctor.

I remembered when my son started hearing things and the doctor said he needed to take medicine to stop hearing things. That doctor didn't explain to me like this doctor did with the tires. He didn't explain to my son either. So when my son stopped the medicine because it made him sleepy and he started hearing those voices again, I didn't make my son take his medicine. Then my son took someone's life because he said the voices told him to do it. Now I can only see my son when the prison visiting hours are happening, and it is a long drive to get there. Maybe that's why I brought the bottle that day. I have a daughter too in the south. She is with my ex-wife but she is not doing well by her. She is not going to school. I have been trying to get her to come live with me so I can get her to go to school. The lawyers send me all kinds of papers to fill out. My girlfriend helps me with those too. Someday I hope my daughter will come to be with me. Maybe that's why I brought the bottle in. I don't want to be paralyzed when my daughter comes to live with me.

Part XIII
Mental Illness and Stigma

Fatalismo

Elain Occil

Milagros is a 50-year-old Puerto Rican woman whose family I met while over the course of 3 months volunteering at a family medicine clinic in South Bronx. She was accompanied by her two teenage daughters, Amparo, 18, and Beatriz, 13, and her grandson Alberto. She had been widowed 8 years ago and had only got insurance because of Medicaid expansion. She suffered from uncontrolled diabetes, obesity, hypertension, and HIV.

But what most impressed me about Milagros were her eyes. As I had walked in that morning, I saw her walking with her cane, supported by her daughter and in obvious agony. I held the door for her and noticed she had stunning bright green eyes framed by deep crow's feet and dark circles. Her thick jet black hair was heavily streaked with gray.

As my preceptor, who had never met Milagros, reviewed the charts, she noticed that Milagros had not been to the clinic in 6 months and had not picked up any of her medications. Her last A1C was 13% and she had gained weight. She could not remember her last pap smear or mammogram. She had no intention of getting a colonoscopy. When asked, she said that she was tired of fighting fate and that what had happened was meant to happen and what will happen was already decided. God had already decided. There was nothing that she could do to get better when she was already dying.

Over 3 months, I encountered Milagros and Beatriz several times, and she told me about her "cursed" life. She and her husband, Sebastian, had emigrated at 18 from their town in Puerto Rico. Milagros had wanted to be a vet and was thinking about going to school. Living at first with her aunt, they had both begun working in a restaurant owned by a friend and had many neighbors. She had gotten pregnant and had a son, Alejandro. Life was hard but family and friends helped.

E. Occil (✉)
Northeast Ohio Medical University, Rootstown, OH, USA
e-mail: eoccil@neomed.edu

When Milagros went back to work, she had problems with a co-worker who "cursed" her and Alejandro died. Milagros could not stop crying. She could not work. She did not go to church and could not think of school. Sebastian began to drink heavily and became physically and verbally abusive. He was unfaithful and had children outside of the marriage, and eventually they separated. They remained so for several years before giving the marriage a second chance, and Milagros had her daughters. Milagros stayed home to take care of the family but visited friends and went to church. They were happy.

Until Sebastian got sick. As he got weaker and weaker, he did not seek medical attention because the family did not have insurance. He instead stayed in the home hiding from neighbors and lying to friends. Milagros took care of him and prayed. He eventually got so weak he could not eat, and they took him to the hospital. Sebastian was diagnosed with HIV and died of AIDS complications. The family confided this to no one and were secretly tested.

Milagros and Amparo had contracted HIV. Again, Milagros could not stop crying. She told us that she was being punished for her misdeeds and she was already dead. Her body stayed behind for her children but only burdened their lives.

"Why take my medication, I'm already dead".

"How could I come to HIV clinic? Then people would know; what would they say?

No one speaks to us because people are suspicious. His family blames me already."

Throughout her lamentation, Beatriz remained still and silent, staring ahead. She was suspended from school because of fighting with other children and truancy. Her mother said that she was a good girl who always helped her, whereas Amparo had invited her boyfriend to live with them.

The last time I saw Milagros, she had begun going to HIV clinic via a 2-hour bus and train ride to avoid recognition. It was difficult to get there because of her weight. On occasion, the family had enough money for a taxi home. She also began taking her other medications for her hypertension and diabetes. She still hid from her neighbors and did not go to church but spoke to her sister over the phone. My preceptor tried to convince her to go to counseling individually or as a family. Beatriz had to repeat eighth grade and had begun to self-harm. Amparo had begun to drink and party heavily, leaving Alberto alone with the family. The counseling center was across the street.

Milagros said, "What will people say?"

Milagros was one of my first patients. I had just finished my interviewing course and was ready to practice my newly gained skills. I was excited despite countless warnings about the area and its reputation as among the poorest districts in the USA. But I had already learned that it is neither a crime nor a sin to be poor and poverty did not diminish one's value. I was ready to do what I was taught. I was ready to provide. I was determined to make a human connection. And I did; I looked at her world-weary eyes, the evidence of her suffering and struggle, and found that there was nothing that could have prepared me for such depths. I have always thought the role of a physician was to not only provide care but to support, to listen, and to want to be supportive, caring, and encouraging. I knew that doctors were someone patients could lean on, but in my naiveté due to my sheltered Long Island upbringing, I did not understand the weight of affliction. Milagros and her family had every negative social determinant of health that I could think of.

Milagros was poor and an immigrant, had little education, and did not speak, read, or write English well. She was a single mother and could not work much due to physical impairment. She suffered from chronic disease and was at high risk for complications. I believed there were some aspects of mental illness at play in her presentation. The neighborhood was unsafe and plagued by gang violence and had little green space, limited transportation in comparison to other areas, and few resources such as supermarkets or hospitals. Her neighbors were friendly but distant, and Milagros had little support outside of her children as the majority of her family lived in Puerto Rico. The community did not have many outreach programs that Milagros participated in, and she had deep-seated and well-founded fears of discrimination. Though Milagros had insurance, the clinic did not have many providers and there was a long waiting list.

To me, the most pressing of her issues was her *fatalismo* or the belief that fate is unchangeable. If something is fated to happen, it will happen, and no preventative measure would fix that. This belief is the antithesis of primary care. When I heard Milagros express these beliefs, I felt an overwhelming sense of danger. This is the patient we lose to follow-up, the patient who has myocardial infarction and major stroke and amputations, the patient who suffers a horrible, painful, and preventable death. *Fatalismo* is more than a cultural belief; it is the culmination of systematic, long-term disengagement due to her enduring social determinants of health.

Yet, during my time with Milagros, I saw her overcome and take steps to improve her health. Though, at the end of my experience, there was still much to address, she had some hope and faith in her ability to take care for the future of her family. What caused me the most distress was Beatrice's worsening mental state. As a developing child, Beatrice had endured the same social milieu that her family did and witnessed the breakdown of her family. In my opinion, she is at most risk and deserving of attention.

Aging Out of Pediatrics

Sunny Dhoopar

It was September of 2017 I started seeing patients in my new job and was excited to meet new patients. I saw a 22-year-old woman, here to establish care, as written on my clinic template. I walked into the room to see this grown-up woman sitting next to a concerned father.

As we started talking, both the father and the patient explained the large medical history and how her pediatrician can no longer see her due to her age.

As we continued to speak, we reviewed her medical history and found her to have diagnoses that included Attention Deficit Disorder (ADD) without hyperactivity, chronic fatigue, and fibromyalgia.

She was taking double the normal dose of stimulants, Selective Serotonin Reuptake Inhibitors (SSRIs), and tramadol for pain control. Both she and her father were concerned that she was starting classes for college, and she wants to go to school, but she needs her medications otherwise, and she is panicking how she will function at school.

As they both looked toward me in hope for help with her medical management, I was terrified to continue her current course of therapy. As we continued to talk, I asked her to go over her history a bit more in detail since I have no idea what has happened in the past. They spoke of an accident close to 10 years ago where she was in a car accident. She states she never got better after that. She has had difficulty with focusing, having body pains and fatigue. While talking to her, it was so difficult to keep her in a linear timeline as she continued to want to talk about the last 6 months and go back to relate her complaints ranging 10 years. Her father also added that he is here for the fact that she forgets much of what the doctor tells her, and they want her management plan to be followed at home. By now almost 30 minutes had passed and I was running behind.

S. Dhoopar (✉)
Summa Health Family Medicine Program-Akron Campus, Akron, OH, USA
e-mail: dhoopara@summahealth.org

© The Author(s) 2019
A. Perzynski et al. (eds.), *Health Disparities*,
https://doi.org/10.1007/978-3-030-12771-8_44

I had her fill out the release of records and brought her back within 1 week for follow-up. I knew that I did not feel safe with the plan she was on. I told her that if I was 22 years old, I would want to be getting a job and an education for a good job and to travel with friends. What does she want from her life? This was the first time I saw her light up. She spoke about how she is going to business school and how her father works for himself, and she wants to have a job where she can run a business. She has friends, and she wants to travel too, and she would like to go to Japan someday. I felt that we were able to partner up here, and we spent more time discussing the goals for school and where she is at now. I agreed to help her find some accommodation by writing a letter to the school, but the plan was that we would work toward graduation. I told her that even though her medications were given by her previous doctor, I do not feel comfortable with her current regimen. She was very scared to be off of these medications, but her father spoke up and said well let's hear your doctor out with his plan. I discussed that with the diagnosis they were presenting with, I would like an adult psychiatrist to evaluate and help with tapering these medications off. I agreed I would not stop them cold. We again spoke about her concerns but with explanation she was agreeable, and I placed a psychiatry consult and refilled her medications.

I saw her again 1 month later, and both her and her father were excited to say they really liked the psychiatrist and his office. She has started counseling and he also recommended tapering off the medications. She was excited to tell me about her school, but she also had 2 days where she missed school due to her fibromyalgia pains. She was hoping to have a letter from me. I asked her how she managed this pain and if it kept her in bed, why she did not call the clinic or have her parents bring her to clinic? She did not think it was needed, but she was in no shape to go to school. I told her that I would not be able to help her unless she is telling me the time she has these flares. That it would be her responsibility. Her father agreed, and I asked her how the accommodation for class selection and seating upfront was taken by the school. She was happy that they were able to provide this. She also told me about how her parents had organized for her to go to Japan over winter break. I encouraged her to keep working hard and that I would see her back in the new year.

While working as the inpatient attending, I noticed my patient's name appears on the emergency department visit roster. Our senior resident was reviewing the charts, and I saw that it was a young adult female, with multiple psychiatric diagnosis who was presenting with dizziness to the emergency room. I saw the whole team roll their eyes and already make up their mind that this was a psychiatric complaint. When I went to the emergency room to staff the admission, she was lying down in a dark room with a towel over her face, and both of her parents were sitting at the bedside. She ran a fever the last week, and for 2 days, she was having nausea and vomiting, and overnight she was week and now very dizzy with any movement. I asked the patient if the light was bothering her and why she needed the towel. She said the light was ok but the towel weight just felt better. I asked her about her visit to Japan and then did a quick physical exam. After this, we discussed keeping her in the hospital overnight and the likelihood of this being a viral illness. Overnight, the mother had become frantic related to her child's health to the point that the resident on-call had to call me to speak to her during the late hours of the night. I reassured her and reviewed the work-up and possible causes of her symptoms. In the morning I saw the mother who was angry and concerned and projecting this to the staff taking care of them. I spent a long while prior to entering the patient's room to listen to the concerns of the staff and residents. I then spent a longer time answering the mother's questions and having the mother take part in the physical exam of the patient. We made a safe plan and then discharged them home.

Judged by Physicians

Stefanie Delvecchio

A 36-year-old Caucasian female with a past history including recurrent major depressive disorder, anxiety, PTSD, unspecified mood disorder, tobacco abuse, and previous rupture of a brain aneurysm (post-surgery with middle cerebral artery stenting in 2012) presented to the office to newly establish care.

When I entered the room, the patient appeared very anxious. She was fidgeting with her hands and pacing around the room. She began the encounter by informing me that she had a 25-year history of daily marijuana use. She stated that marijuana was the only thing that ever helped to control her anxiety. She informed me that she has struggled with physical abuse and domestic violence her entire life. She added that for a period of time, many years ago, she had been raped by multiple different men. She has difficulty trusting people.

The patient's husband was recently sent to jail, because a man in her building called the police stating that her husband was physically abusing her. She stated that the man was lying and trying to hurt her family, but could not identify why. She added that her husband has always been good to her and that she is unable to function mentally or physically without his care. She has been trying to get him released from jail but stated that no one listens to her. The patient requested documentation from our office requesting his release (because he is her primary caregiver). She also requested a prescription for Ativan to help manage her anxiety, because her husband had been supplying her marijuana, and she had been without it since his time of arrest. She has had bad experiences with doctors in the past, which she attributes to her poverty and a generalized lack of insight into her struggles. She often feels judged by physicians.

The patient has two young boys at home. She worries about her family's safety every day. She informed me that there is a man in the building who has a gun and is constantly threatening to harm her and her family but that the police won't do

S. Delvecchio (✉)
Family Medicine Residency, Summa Health System/Barberton Campus, Northeast, OH, USA
e-mail: delvecchios@summahealth.org

© The Author(s) 2019
A. Perzynski et al. (eds.), *Health Disparities*,
https://doi.org/10.1007/978-3-030-12771-8_45

anything to help. Her family doesn't currently have the resources to move to a safer neighborhood. She is anxious all the time and worries that her children are seeing her this way. She wishes to be a better role model for her kids. I asked the patient if she would be willing to pursue counseling. She told me that she has been to counseling for most of her life but "graduated" from it, because her therapists told her that she was too self-motivated and successful in achieving her therapeutic goals. She doesn't believe that therapy is helpful and refuses to be referred for counseling again at this time. She is not currently on any psychiatric medications.

Ugh

Sladjana Courson

Ugh. I am ashamed to say that is the first word that comes to my mind when I see Jake's name on my schedule for the day. He is 10 and he has been my patient since he was born. He has an 8-year-old sister Annie and a 5-year-old brother Jimmy. They usually all come in together with their mother even if only one of them has an appointment that day. They all have a variety of mental health diagnoses, including ADHD, OCD, and PTSD, and Jake also has autism. It has not been easy to align him with mental health providers. I have tried to help mom deal with his aggressive behaviors—the hitting, biting, and yelling—but I feel that I have failed them on several occasions. Mom tries her best, but she has some cognitive delays herself and doesn't always know how to handle him. Regularly they are in the emergency room where he is given medications to sedate him, and then they are then sent home. They come to their appointment with me and I feel helpless. How do I get this family all the assistance and guidance they need?

S. Courson (✉)
Akron Children's Hospital, Akron, OH, USA

Northeast Ohio Medical University, Rootstown, OH, USA
e-mail: scourson@akronchildrens.org

© The Author(s) 2019
A. Perzynski et al. (eds.), *Health Disparities*,
https://doi.org/10.1007/978-3-030-12771-8_46

Will You Be My PCP?

Adefunke Adedipe

I was running 20 minutes late and I was preparing for the worst: a patient sitting there, irritated that I had not arrived on time. As I opened the door, the first thing I noticed was the patient curled up on the examination table with a blanket covered over her head.

When I asked the patient what brought her into the office today, she stated that she feared she was pregnant and had some abdominal pain. As per normal routine, I did a thorough history and physical and gynecological examination. When I was done, I told her my plan and that I would have the attending come in shortly. As I closed the curtains to allow her to dress up, the patient muttered asking if she could "see someone to talk to." When asking further, the patient stated that she had been depressed for some years but had worsened within the last month. I tried to delve in more in regard to her depression, but the patient felt uncomfortable and would not talk anymore. I thought at this time it was best for me to precept with the attending.

When the attending arrived to the room and spoke to the patient about her depression, the patient started to break down and cry. She stated that her best friend was killed 1 month ago by a man she knew, and she was having a hard time coping. She stated that 1 month ago, she tried to kill herself with pills. She also stated that if her pregnancy test was positive she would have gone home and "completed the job." When asked if she had a safe place to go, she stated that she was homeless for the past month and had no family or friends. As I talked with her some more, I thought it was best for her to go to the emergency department (ED) for further evaluation. Before I walked her down to the ED, the patient stated that this was the first time she ever had the opportunity to tell someone what she was going through.

When she said that to me, I couldn't help but to think about how her depression could have been missed. While I did detailed history and examination on the patient,

A. Adedipe (✉)
Department of Family Medicine, The MetroHealth System, Cleveland, OH, USA
e-mail: aadedipe@metrohealth.org

© The Author(s) 2019
A. Perzynski et al. (eds.), *Health Disparities*,
https://doi.org/10.1007/978-3-030-12771-8_47

it wasn't until the end that I knew she really wanted help with her depression. What was comforting to me was that she wanted me to be her primary care provider (PCP) and begged me never to leave her side. I told her that I would love to be her PCP and that I would want her to follow up in a week to see how she was doing. I followed her stay at the ED, but it looked like she left against medical advice (AMA) and refused to have further evaluation. I tried calling the patient several times but the line never went through.

As I look back to this encounter, I really questioned whether or not this patient would follow up. Here was a patient who was severely depressed and homeless and had no meaningful connections at this point in her life. I really hope she follows up.

Part XIV
Insurance

My Lucky Twins

Sheng Liu

I was in the USA for only 8 months when I found myself pregnant. It was not a surprise because I could not afford any birth control. I was working in a Chinese restaurant at the time. I had no money and I had no insurance. I have not seen any doctor since I came to the USA. My husband and most of his family had not seen anyone either. Although they said there was a Chinese-speaking doctor who worked in Chinatown clinic, I did not have to go to see anyone and none of my family had met her.

I waited as long as possible because they said that seeing doctors in the USA was very expensive. My pregnancy started showing. My coworkers started asking questions. So finally I went to the clinic in the location according to my friend. I encountered the people from that clinic. The girl at front desk spoke Toishanese, Cantonese, and Mandarin. My anxiety was a lot less after talking to her.

I was still anxious about how much I had to pay. Depending on how much I could afford, I was going to decide how often I would visit the doctor. I saw a different girl and showed her all the paper works she wanted. I had very little money in my bank, and I made very little at work. At the end of the visit, she gave me a piece of paper saying a number "6" on it. She said that I did not have to pay for the visits with this doctor and all the doctors in the hospital. The only thing I had to pay was for the medication. It was like I had meat pies coming down from the sky. I did not have to pay for my baby's visit. But nothing good came cheap. Was this doctor good enough for my pregnancy? Was she seeing me for free because she was not a worthy doctor? But they said she was good.

With some doubt, I finally met this Chinese-speaking doctor. She looked friendly. She speaks Mandarin, while I speak Toishanese and some Mandarin. We communicated pretty well. She did not look young enough to be the type of doctors who just

S. Liu (✉)
The MetroHealth System, Asian Services in Action, Inc., Cleveland, OH, USA
e-mail: sliu@metrohealth.org

© The Author(s) 2019
A. Perzynski et al. (eds.), *Health Disparities*,
https://doi.org/10.1007/978-3-030-12771-8_48

came out of school and had no experience. She told me she had worked for Metro Hospital for 15 years and she had been mainly working at the main hospital. So I decided to trust her.

Soon I found that I had twins. I was nervous but happy. After all there were no twins in my family since my uncle Yang. I did not know what to expect from now on. My doctor referred me to a high-risk specialist. But I could not understand him well because he could not find any Toishanese to do a phone translation. I had to settle with a Cantonese translator. Every time I saw him, I returned to my doctor for more explanation.

I was getting a lot of ultrasound. Time went by. I was told my babies were growing fine and equally (which was important according to my doctor) and I had two boys. Then my doctor called 1 day after a regular ultrasound. She told me to see the high-risk guy right away. I knew something was wrong.

I was terrified when he told me that there was a condition called twin-to-twin transfusion. I had to have a procedure done to cut off the connection between my twins. If not I might lose both of them. I may still lose both of them if the procedure did not go well.

I did not have insurance. I was not able to get government insurance because I was not a citizen. Metro rated me based on my income as a waitress. All of my care was free at that time. But the procedure the doctor was saying was not available at Metro. I had to go to from Cleveland all the way to Cincinnati for this procedure. There was no option like rating available at the Children's Hospital in Cincinnati because it was not a county hospital like Metro. I had to pay a lot of money for this procedure.

I came to the USA only for little over a year at the time. My husband was working but between him and I, we were making US$1500 a month. We had an 8-year-old daughter. I had to think about her. She needed her own home. We would never be able to pay back the hundreds of thousands of dollars the procedure might cost me. What would my daughter do if we do not even have the money for her to go to college? Her life would be ruined because of us as her parents.

What if the surgery did not go well? Then we would have spent a lot of money for nothing and still won't be able to save my twins. Would it be more feasible to travel back to China for this procedure? I did not think the procedure was available even in the state capital Guangzhou. I might have to go to the capital city Beijing. Was it safe to travel in my stage of pregnancy? Could I get back in China on time?

I started to lose sleep and could not feel happy any more. I started making mistakes and almost got myself fired from my job. My twins were precious to me but so was my daughter. I was about to lose them because we could not afford the surgery. Or I would have made everyone in my family suffer the financial consequences by having the surgery. My husband and I and his family spent a lot of time arguing, and in the end, I was more upset.

I did not show up for my appointment and my doctor called me finally. She said not to worry about the cost and to save the twins first. I had not much time before both twins' condition got much worse. One twin could get too small because the blood was stolen away by the other. He could suffer heart failure because of his blood being too low. The other twin could also suffer from having too much blood. When both had problems with their hearts, it would be too late to do anything. My doctor said that it was okay to worry about paying for it later. There would be something I could do after the babies were born. I was appreciative but really did not think that she could relay my concerns with her doctor's salary. (They said that all doctors make a lot of money.)

Sensing that I was still having trouble making up my mind, she said she would call me later. She told me to go online to explore the options and try to use the dictionary or something to find out what I was looking for.

Luckily I was better with written English than speaking it. I could recognize a decent number of words. I spent most of my time trying to read some information about the surgery. The Internet said that Cincinnati Children's Hospital had a good track record of this surgery. The success rate was good. The bad result was not too much. I gained a lot more confidence by reading through the materials, even though I was only half understanding it. My husband and I finally decided to move forward with the procedure. We were quickly scheduled with the doctor in Cincinnati Hospital. We drove down and talked to the two doctors there, where one was an Indian doctor and the other a Malaysian. They both were very nice and patient.

After that meeting we were asked to return on the following Monday for the scheduled surgery. On the surgery date, my husband and I got up at 3 am to drive to Cincinnati and arrived early to the hospital. (That would save 1 day of hotel expense.) I went through the surgery without much memory. It was like a dream. When it was over, the doctors told us that they were happy with the result. We were happy too besides the overshadow of worries that we possibly just generated a huge bill that could potentially ruin our lives for years to come.

Shortly after the surgery we were moved to an adult hospital where the hospital room was cheaper. After 2–3 days we were back home. I had more ultrasound tests. And the difference in my twins' weight did not change but did not get worse either. We were so glad and so worried at the same time. At that time the partial bill from Children's Hospital for the surgery alone was well over US$40,000. We shared this with my doctor at the visit.

Then my doctor called to ask me for my permission to send out an *Ask for Help* email. She said she would like to see if it was okay to disclose some information about my twins for me to receive donation. She said she wouldn't need to disclose my name or address but the story needed to go out. I said to her that I had to talk to my husband and his family.

I had a conversation with my husband and his parents. The Chinese people live in such a tight circle in Chinatown that everyone knows everyone. People would be able to figure out it was us who needed help for having twins. We would lose face because we couldn't even afford having babies. That was too much insult to realize if people recognize us, and they were bound to figure out. There would be too much gossip for my husband's family who had resided in Chinatown for a long time. I told my doctor "no" when she called back. I knew she was puzzled but accepted what I said.

We were under the shadow of burden of the hospital debt for a few months. Whatever was to come would come. I might as well not worry about it right now. My twins need to be fed and cared for. Like my doctor said, I would worry about the bill when it was here.

But the dreadful bill collection never came. The social worker in Children's Hospital learned about my struggles and helped me file a piece of paper. We finally needed to pay US$2000 for the whole thing. To this date I am still worried that would be a big mistake. Now my twins are 3 years old. The bill still has not come so I think we are safe. Every time I play with my 3-year-old twins, I feel very lucky. Lives don't come that easily. Life in the USA is so strange and alien to me, at least in the beginning. Now it is a little bit better. It is terrifying to be sick in the USA. I got away this time, and I may not be that lucky next time.

What Kind of System Is This?

Betsy Ekey

As a physician assistant in an occupational medicine clinic, I frequently encountered patients who needed to be referred to their primary care provider for the evaluation of non-work-related diseases and disorders. As a medical provider, I was capable of evaluating and treating a patient for things like hypertension or diabetes, but the treatment was beyond the scope of the practice, so patient education and guidance to their primary care provider were key.

The patient population was typically between the ages of 18 and 65 years and patients were sent to the clinic for evaluation without needing to pay for services. The employer's worker's compensation insurance coverage or the employer was responsible for the payment as long as the care was given for an issue that arose due to work or from their work. Frequently, the medical care given was the only care that patient would receive since worker's compensation coverage or employer payment for occupational illness/injuries did not guarantee that the patient had private health insurance or that they could afford health care.

Occasionally, a patient would seek care for something that they believed must be a work-related illness or injury, and I would deem it not related to work. Even though it was not related to work, that did not mean that the patient did not need further evaluation and care. One specific patient sought care for testicular swelling that he noticed after lifting heavy boxes. The 24-year-old patient was non-English speaking and was brought to the clinic by his employer. Through an interpreter, a complete history was obtained about his chief complaint. The patient noticed this swelling after lifting heavy boxes, but he did not have any abdominal pain, testicular pain, testicular redness, fever, penile discharge, or difficulty with his urination. Prior to the physical exam, I was starting to develop my list of differential diagnoses and testicular cancer kept entering my mind in addition to inguinal hernia, hydrocele,

B. Ekey, MPAS, PA-C (✉)
Physician Assistant Studies Program, University of Mount Union, Alliance, OH, USA
e-mail: ekeybd@mountunion.edu

© The Author(s) 2019
A. Perzynski et al. (eds.), *Health Disparities*,
https://doi.org/10.1007/978-3-030-12771-8_49

varicocele, or spermatocele. Since he was not having pain, it was less likely that he would have testicular torsion, epididymitis, or orchitis. My differential diagnosis included only one diagnosis (inguinal hernia) that would be work related.

The physical examination confirmed that the patient had a scrotal mass that did not transilluminate and no inguinal hernia. Testicular cancer again landed at the top of my differential diagnosis list. How best to address this suspected testicular cancer in a non-English speaking patient who is in an occupational medicine clinic and who does not understand that in the United States, not all clinics take care of every health issue? The employer's worker's compensation insurer would not pay for further evaluation of a scrotal mass but this patient clearly needed an ultrasound. If I ordered the ultrasound, the patient would receive the bill, but as a medical provider with this "must not miss" diagnosis, I wanted to ensure that this patient not only got an ultrasound but was not lost to follow-up. Through the interpreter, I tried to explain my concerns and give the patient resources for further evaluation at the health system's primary care clinic in order to get the ultrasound but the patient got angry that this was not considered work related and he thought his employer should pay. Was this all lost in translation? What kind of system do I work in that cannot get a patient the care that they need? Would this suspected cancer advance and spread because the patient doesn't trust the system based on his interaction with me?

The Fall That Won't Stop Falling

Sarah Shick

The brakes of my dark green Honda Accord squeaked as my boyfriend eased his way down the steep concrete hill leading to the cavernous loading bay for the hospital's emergency department. It seemed ironic to me that a place for the sickest people would smell like exhaust fumes, motor oil, and cigarette smoke.

A tall, slender young man jumped up from the valet station and ran to open the door for me, asking if we would like to take advantage of the complimentary valet parking for patients. My waist length hair was still done up from the wedding we attended the night before, but my reflection in the automatic doors showed a frightening lack of color except for the dark, sunken eyes staring back at me. I normally walked with a cane, but I was so weak that I readily accepted a wheelchair ride to the triage station.

Walking with a switch in her hips, a woman with curly hair and purple eye shadow to match the characters on her scrubs entered the lobby to call my name and wheel me into a little office. While she checked my vital signs, she asked me, "So, honey, what brings you in here this lovely day?"

"Um… I've been throwing up blood since yesterday, and when I called my doctor today he kind of lost it and told me to get my butt in here," I replied sheepishly.

The nurse's eyes grew large and she shook her head, "For how long? Honey, that's not good. You should know, you should never come in to an emergency department and tell them that you're throwing up blood because the most unpleasant experiences are sure to follow. I'm going to tell you now so you can prepare yourself—they will be shoving a tube up through your nose down through to your stomach. But don't worry, though, they'll use some lube," she said, chuckling to herself. "Now it says here that you're a Workers' Comp. patient, is that right? You can't be throwing up blood from work. What is your other insurance?"

S. Shick (✉)
Department of Sociology, Case Western Reserve University, Center for Health Care Research and Policy, The MetroHealth System, Cleveland, OH, USA
e-mail: ses165@case.edu

"This *is* from my Workers' Comp. claim. I don't have any other insurance. I fell through a trapdoor, hit the top stairs so hard that I flew up out of it, then gravity pulled me back down and I kept falling down the flight of steps, bouncing up and down until the momentum flung me face-first onto a concrete floor. I almost died. The doctors have had me on a lot of medications and my main doc was worried that it might have caused this stomach bleeding," I explained, growing frustrated with her line of questioning.

The receptionist gave my boyfriend the same lecture; it was clear to us that she and the nurse assumed we were trying to cheat the system. We were both multiracial: with his long dreadlocks, he was often told he resembled Bob Marley with slightly lighter skin, and I'd lost count of how many children genuinely believed I was Pocahontas. We wondered if our skin tone factored in to their suspicions, but we decided to give them the benefit of the doubt. By the time I was given a room and the initial tests were completed, and my insurance had been questioned by nearly every physician and nurse we encountered, my boyfriend seemed as if he was going to snap.

He turned to me, his face reddened, and grumbled "I don't get this, you were working your job, you got hurt, we all pay into the system, and yet you have already been to court three times in the last three months to get them to cover your care and pay you the money you were owed. I am sure that the owner of the bar isn't facing the same level of hassle that we are, and he's the one who didn't fix that trapdoor after five other people fell into it in the last three years! And that's not even considering how much you've been suffering. You looked like a Star Wars Storm Trooper in your neck brace and body brace the first month after breaking your darn back."

I tended to be passive and patient, especially when I was very sick or in pain, so my boyfriend became a fierce advocate. I frequently caught him shaking his head in sheer disbelief at the bureaucracy and judgment we faced from people who saw me as nothing more than either a potential unpaid medical bill, a criminal, or a hypochondriac.

I would joke with him during these times, trying to meet the humiliation with wry humor, "As if there were some appeal to trading my day job with a world-renowned event planner, a $250 a night gig moonlighting as a bartender and booking agent, just to start faking a brain injury, some fractured bones, and spinal cord damage. Hey, you know my acting skills needed a brush up, anyway, right? Yup, and who wouldn't trade all that to fake an injury for less than $600 a month, five days a week of exhausting medical encounters, body braces, a walker fit for a nursing home, a loss of my identity, loss of my social network, and constant disorienting pain. That's perfectly logical… at least according Workers' Comp. and these doctors, and they're obviously *way* better educated than us, right?" Sometimes I could make him laugh, but sometimes it was all just too much.

Eventually, three nurses and a doctor came in and sat at my bed at an upright angle. The room began shrinking as they laid out the blue paper cloth, opened plastic tubing from its sterile packaging, and began to lube it up. Two nurses stood at either side and held my shoulders while the third nurse stood behind my head. The doctor, a slightly uneasy, heavyset Middle Eastern man instructed me, "Alright, this is going to go better for everyone if you just work with us. We're going to put this to through your nose and into your stomach. Your body will want to fight it, but you just have to keep swallowing. If you don't cooperate with us it's going to make it more uncomfortable for you."

The two nurses on either side of me held my shoulders against the hospital bed and the third nurse held my head in place. The resident balanced his hand against my lower jaw while he started to shove the tube into my nose. I tried to be strong and hold back the urge to cry, but it was as if my body decided to release independent of my emotions or choice, and the tears gushed down my cheeks in two salty rivers of anguish. At first the tube was slightly cooler than my body and it scratched as it traveled through me, deeper and deeper until I felt it touch the top of my throat. I gagged and reflexively tried to grab the tube, but the nurses swiftly pinned down my arms. My spine and right hip, which were still healing from fractures, began a searing protest to the tension and positioning. I felt primal, like a cornered animal, but simultaneously found strange comfort in nostalgic flashbacks to childhood and being forced to take what I used to call "the bad medicine," which was never anything worse than Children's Tylenol or antibiotics to help me feel better.

One of the nurses and my boyfriend tried to offer words of comfort, but I could barely hear them over my body's screaming reaction. After what seemed like 20 minutes, they completed their testing and said casually, "All right, get ready. This is going to feel weird but it's going to come out really quickly." Like a mechanic pulling the dipstick to check my oil levels, the resident nonchalantly pulled the tube, giving me a whole new concept of nausea that felt like my stomach was being pulled up through my throat into my nose and out of me with a burning, violating slickness.

When they left the room, I turned to my boyfriend, with tears still streaming down my face, trembling while holding a tissue against my lightly bleeding nose, and said, "I feel like I just got nose raped. That was one of the worst experiences of my life."

"No offense, but that was one of the worst experiences of my life, too. Well, the nurse warned you. This will teach you not to fake things to cheat the system." He laughed, and rolled his eyes, then gave me a kiss on the forehead. I thanked him for his support.

About an hour or two later, the resident walked in with a spring in his step, and said, "I've got two bits of good news for you. First, the blood we found in your stomach was dark brown, so it looks like the bleed has stopped on its own and we won't have to do any surgery. Second, congratulations, you're pregnant."

"That's impossible, I have endometriosis. I've been told I won't be able to have kids. I tried to get pregnant for years, and eventually the doctors told me I'm infertile. There must be a mistake, please do the test again." I said, half laughing, sure that there was some simple medical error.

Three pregnancy tests later, the results were confirmed, and one of the nurses kindly said, "Miracles happen, darling. Guess you are just meant to be a mom." I went through the next weeks feeling elated about this unexpected blessing, with my sisters and parents thrilled that I would be starting the next generation. Everything was going well until my third OB appointment, and second ultrasound. They rushed around with pursed lips, and no one would look me in the eye. Over the next three days my pregnancy slowly ended. I was eventually hospitalized and only narrowly avoided surgery from complications. The doctors told me that the recent trauma from falling through the trapdoor, and the stomach bleed from the medications I was prescribed afterward, caused my body to be too weak to maintain a pregnancy.

Who knew that working three jobs to pay student loans so I could afford to finish my degree, a careless owner disregarding a major safety hazard despite watching other people get hurt, and taking medications that were supposed to help me heal, would take away the one chance I had at becoming a mother? I struggled for months to overcome the depression that followed. Eventually, I learned to treat it as a metaphor, instead "giving birth" to a new version of myself, as a woman with a disability and a deep passion to help improve the world for people like me.

Part XV
Fragmented Care

I'm Going to Be OK

Emily Godlewski

"It's about time you got in here."

I was just a few minutes late getting started for Kathleen's appointment, so it seemed apparent she was in a hurry. Kathleen sat in a chair next to our examination table. She was restless and her excess body weight poured around the arm rests. I politely explained that I had spent the last few moments reading over her records.

Last night, Kathleen had been to the emergency department because of a severe headache, with characteristics and intensity unlike any she'd had in the past. She felt a deep throbbing behind and around her right eye that radiated to her temple and forehead. The emergency physicians did two different images of her brain—a CT scan and a CT angiogram—to see whether she was having a stroke. They also drew bloodwork and gave her some morphine to help with the pain. By the time the brain imaging was completed and reviewed, her headache had greatly improved.

At today's visit, Kathleen told me the emergency physician said her imaging and blood work were "fine," but that she needed to see her primary care physician right away. So, here she was, sitting in my office, begrudgingly. Her headache had not returned and she had no other physical complaints. I asked a few questions to confirm the details of the headache symptoms she had the day before. Then I asked what she thought had caused her headache. Kathleen essentially thought that yesterday's headache was a chance occurrence. And, although she was worried it might Re-occur, she felt there was no need to further discuss the matter.

I gently explained, "Well, Kathleen, I'm a bit concerned about what happened yesterday… (brief pause) …Your blood work showed an abnormality in something called the erythrocyte sedimentation rate, or ESR. Because of this I am worried you might have a condition called temporal arteritis."

E. Godlewski, MD (✉)
Aultman Hospital Family Medicine Residency Program/Northeast Ohio Medical University, Canton, OH, USA
e-mail: Emily.Godlewski@aultman.com

© The Author(s) 2019
A. Perzynski et al. (eds.), *Health Disparities*,
https://doi.org/10.1007/978-3-030-12771-8_51

169

Usually, I would pause here to allow the patient to ask questions, so we could discuss what temporal arteritis was. With Kathleen, however, I knew she would cut me off at any moment. I knew I was dumping a lot of info on to her, but I had learned from experience that each small suggestion would be met with a strong reaction. Thus, I quickly spit out my recommendations: "I would like to draw more blood work today. We also may need to have you see a specialist so that he or she can do a small biopsy from your forehead, where the headache was bothering you. And, if the headache comes back, we may need to start you on a type of medication called a steroid. What questions can I…".

Her response was abrupt and animated, "I ain't going to hear that."

"What part is hard for you to hear?"

"You ain't telling me that."

"How are you feeling about this information?"

At first, she had no further response. The silence was uncomfortable and several times I fumbled over my words, trying to figure out how best to connect with her.

Kathleen told me several more times that she wasn't "going to hear that."

I apologized. It seemed obvious she did not expect to hear bad news at this visit based on her interpretation of her emergency department visit the night before.

I'd known Kathleen for 6 months. During that time, I'd had to disclose several pieces of disheartening news to her: Her diabetes was poorly controlled, evidenced by a very elevated hemoglobin A1c. She'd recently had a recurrence of atrial fibrillation that necessitated the initiation of blood thinners, which can have risky side effects. Her brain scans indicated that she had likely had many small strokes. And, her Carotid arteries were significantly narrowed, so we agreed that she should be taking a medication to lower her cholesterol called a statin, which would also decrease the narrowing of her Carotid arteries and decrease her risk of another stroke.

Kathleen had also been to see two specialists over the past few months: When she joined my practice, she was already seeing an endocrinologist. One afternoon I was notified by his office that Kathleen had missed two appointments. I contacted her to ask what had happened and she explained that she didn't feel her diabetes was a problem. I tried to explain that her hemoglobin A1c was very elevated, indicating that her diabetes was indeed a problem. She seemed genuinely surprised that her diabetes was poorly controlled, as though this was never explained to her. She had also seen a cardiologist in the past, who apparently told her that she no longer needed blood thinners because her atrial fibrillation had been corrected. Unfortunately, it had now recurred, so I recommended that she consider restarting a blood thinner. She was very frustrated by this change in recommended treatment. In both instances, Kathleen's frustration with the overall situation was directed towards me.

Her response to my suggestions today was not a surprise, "I'm tired of going to all you doctors. I see one doctor here and you send me to another doctor there."

In my heart, I knew that the idea of possible temporal arteritis would be difficult for her to entertain. I am not sure how long it had been since Kathleen had optimal health, but it surely was months—even years—before we met. I do not know what messages she'd received in the past—about her vascular disease, the risks of poorly controlled diabetes, or of the toll that obesity was taking on her body. And I am not sure whether her recent spate of new diagnoses truly represented a rapid decline, a fresh perspective from a new physician, or simply reflected the realities of her chronic conditions.

It seems like each time I see Kathleen, the bad news outpaces her acceptance of traditional therapies.

"I'm going to be ok," Kathleen told me.

I briefly wondered whose convincing whom of this, before I decided to pivot back to her treatment options.

It was futile. Kathleen's mind was made up and she repeated: "I'm going to be ok."

She Smiles

Hemalatha Senthilkumar

Ms. B is a 48-year-old patient who has been visiting Family Medicine clinic since 2008. I first started caring for her in 2010. She was seeing me for her blood pressure which has been difficult to control. Lack of medical insurance has played a role as well as side effects to medications. She is taking only one of the three medications prescribed for her blood pressure. The one thing she is careful about is watching her salt intake. We both discuss and come up with a plan for her blood pressure and she agrees to follow up. I see her one more time and then she is lost for follow-up. I forget about her.

A year later, the clinic case coordinator KE informs me that Ms. B will be seeing me for a post-stroke follow-up visit. She was treated for a stroke at another hospital, in a different local health system. Meanwhile, she has also developed diabetes. Ms. B keeps her appointment with me. She tells me she lost her medical insurance and was unable to come see me for quite some time, but now she has coverage through the hospital's pro-rated insurance coverage program. The stroke has left her with numbness in her hands, but she has recovered from the facial and left upper extremity weakness. She leaves the clinic promising to follow back. A few weeks later KE informs me that Ms. B developed blood clots in her leg and was treated at another hospital and I will be seeing her shortly.

Ms. B keeps her appointment. She tells me she developed deep vein thrombosis. She has a venous filter placed to prevent a blood clot from travelling to her lungs. She was told she was not a candidate for blood thinners due to recent history of stroke and the risk of bleeding in her brain. She was also told her filter needs to be removed in 6 months. I notice her blood pressure is elevated, and she informs me her blood pressure medications were changed in the outside hospital. I make note of the changes, request outside records, and make some adjustment in her blood pressure

H. Senthilkumar (✉)
Department of Family Medicine, The MetroHealth System, Case Western Reserve University, Cleveland, OH, USA
e-mail: hsenthilkumar@metrohealth.org

© The Author(s) 2019
A. Perzynski et al. (eds.), *Health Disparities*,
https://doi.org/10.1007/978-3-030-12771-8_52

medication. Ms. B raises a concern regarding her heavy monthly bleeding. We decide to get pelvic ultrasound and check her blood. The ultrasound shows a benign uterine tumor called fibroid which is the cause of her heavy monthly bleeding. The blood test reveals anemia and I start her on iron pills. I refer her to see an OB/GYN and ask her to keep me posted. Ms. B returns and informs me that the OB/GYN determined she is not a candidate for hysterectomy. They have told her to see intervention radiology for a radiation procedure which will be noninvasive.

Meanwhile she continues to have heavy monthly bleeding. She is asked by radiology to get an MRI before she can have the procedure. Her blood pressure is in better control but still above normal. She tells me there is a lot going on. She states she is taking her medication. I get her blood count checked. Ms. B returns earlier than expected to discuss her MRI. I already knew her results. Ms. B has a kidney mass detected incidentally when she gets her MRI and she is here to talk with me regarding this. I tell her she will need to see urology and KE makes her appointment. I arrange for blood transfusion as her counts have dropped further.

In a few weeks, I see Ms. B for a follow-up. She tells me she had a partial nephrectomy for renal cell carcinoma. The urologist is optimistic, as the cancer has been removed completely. I tell her I am happy for her and she is lucky to have survived both a stroke and cancer. The only issue now is her monthly bleeding. Her blood pressure is in good control. Ms. B gets another blood transfusion, and later her OB/GYN performs the hysterectomy. Meanwhile, her filter is also removed. This time when I see Ms. B, I tell her she has no more troubles in her way. Everything seems to be looking good. I congratulate her patience and tell her I am very proud of her.

I was surprised to see MS. B on my schedule earlier then I had planned. Ms. B tells me she was seen in outside hospital for "shakes." She was told it was due to her blood pressure. Changes were made in her blood pressure medication while in the outside hospital. Her blood pressure is mildly elevated today. Her story did not make sense, and I tell her she will need to get a test called EEG and see neurology as I am concerned for seizures. Before she sees neurology, I learn from the emergency department that she is admitted in the hospital for seizures and she is started on medication. The cause of seizures is her stroke. KE makes a follow-up appointment and I see Ms. B again. She tells me she is anxious and afraid. She is now living with her daughter. She is scared to live alone. I inform her that the blood test shows her seizure medication dose needs to be reduced. She requests no dose change, she would rather take a higher dose of seizure medication than to suffer another seizure. I agree but advise her to see her neurologist as well and to have a discussion with him. This visit was difficult for me. I could understand her stress and suffering she is going through. I offer words of encouragement. I praised her suggestion regarding her seizure medication and tell her it is a smart idea to stay with her daughter.

A few weeks later, it was as usual a busy clinic day. I received a staff message from KE that Ms. B was told to go to the emergency room. A few hours later, KE sends another message that Ms. B is being transported by life flight to another hospital for emergency surgery. I stop what I am doing. I look through the emergency room visit notes. What is her problem? I just saw her, blood pressure was great, what else can be wrong? I could not believe with what emergency finds. I just freeze and keep staring at the computer. She has acute dissection of aorta. My goodness! This is a real medical emergency! She is being taken by life flight helicopter to another hospital.

This is it. I cannot take this any longer. I leave the clinic and walk straight to KE office. She is on the phone. I wait. I have spoken with KE on several occasions about Ms. B. She is my connection to Ms. B. KE tells me Ms. B is having surgery at this moment. I ask her what happened. KE tells she was having chest pain and given her medical history she was told "just go to ER." I share my dismay with KE about the multiple medical issues Ms. B has been having and how even at the recent visit she was looking great. I recall telling KE, "I will be done and ready to leave this earth if it were me." I also remark that Ms. B will probably not see me again. KE reassures me stating I am a good physician and I have done my best for her. I leave with a heavy heart. All I wanted to do was to read about aortic dissection. It will have to wait as I was running behind in clinic. I will be lucky if I can have lunch. Later I read about aortic dissection. I go through Ms. B's chart to whether there might have been any indicators for aortic dissection other than hypertension and do not find anything.

I was nervous to see Ms. B again. KE had made the follow-up appointment. I was glad she was alive. I was also feeling guilty. Somehow I feel responsible but do not know how. I ask her how she has been. She tells me she is well. She tells me she was operated within 3 hours after being seen in the emergency room. I shudder thinking what if it turned the other way. She has no pain and even stopped taking her pain medication. I ask her if I can see her scar. She shows me and I am relieved. The surgical scar looks beautiful, well healed and I am happy for her. This time I make sure I do not tell her she will have no more problems. I tell her she is a courageous woman. She smiles. She has beat all odds and she knows it.

Bakit? (Why?)

Mariquita Tolentino-Belen

Tan olive skin, wide smile, black hair, dark almond-shaped eyes, short and thin, mid 40s… a very typical person I used to see while I was in medical school. I see such patients less often now in private practice.

Why is she so familiar? She is a Filipino like me! That in itself gave us an instant connection. It is as if I've known her forever.

She came to establish care. First visit on a cold February morning. She has been seen in the emergency room 3 months ago due to abdominal pain. No workup was done and was advised to follow up with primary care provider (PCP).

But she has no PCP. She just arrived from the Philippines. She called the new patient coordinator and was told that a Filipina doctor is available but it will be 3 months wait. She patiently waited for that day.

That February morning, she was very frail. She has past history of ovarian cancer that she underwent total hysterectomy and oophorectomy 10 years ago. She has a palpable fist-size mass on the suprapubic area. She lost weight significantly, more than 20 pounds in 3 months. She lost her appetite.

I sent her for STAT CT abdomen and blood work. It revealed the mass is a likely malignancy. I called the oncologist and surgeon to facilitate care. They offered outpatient follow-up and did not accept her for direct admission. I begged… they said, "Come to the ED if she crashes." Those were the specific words they said to me.

She deteriorated so fast; she developed obstructive nephropathy secondary to the mass. She was not able to eat, drink, or even urinate. She suffered for days and yet did not go to the emergency room. She was afraid that she will be sent home again. She lived through the pain as long as she could.

When she decompensated, her sister-in-law who is a nurse and a Caucasian had to force her to come in to the emergency room. She was admitted in the intensive

M. Tolentino-Belen (✉)
Aultman Hospital-Northeast Ohio Medical University, Canton, OH, USA
e-mail: 5955@aultman.com

© The Author(s) 2019
A. Perzynski et al. (eds.), *Health Disparities*,
https://doi.org/10.1007/978-3-030-12771-8_53

care unit. I saw her with nephrostomy tube. She is scheduled for surgery. A few months later she died.

Why? When she had abdominal pain at the ED, she was not taken seriously. She never bothered to come back. She was afraid they would not do anything again.

Why? She was not advised about the urgency of establishing with a PCP. Three months is too long. Did the ED doctor even touch her abdomen? She is so thin. That mass can be felt even by a person without any formal medical training.

Why me? Could she not have been seen sooner by a PCP who has an earlier opening?

Why? If I were white, would they have accepted her right away for direct admission? Would they have treated her urgently?

I still have so many questions. *Bakit? Bakit? Bakit?* Health care disparities does not only apply to patients. I see it, I feel it, I live it.

Part XVI
Workshop, Activity and Facilitator Resources

Guidelines for Health Disparities Case Narratives Workshops

Adam Perzynski and Ifeolorunbode Adebambo

Overview

Health disparities encompass ongoing inequality in environments, access to care, healthcare quality, and health outcomes experienced by racial/ethnic minorities, persons of low socioeconomic status, and other disadvantaged or vulnerable groups. The Centers for Disease Control and Prevention (CDC) has primary goals of reducing preventable morbidity and mortality and eliminating disparities in health between segments of the US population. (1) Increasing awareness among providers is a necessary step in eliminating health disparities, yet changes in attitudes are needed in order to change behaviors (2). The use of case narratives is a familiar approach in medical education (3, 4), but case narratives have not been routinely used for learning about health disparities. We will model and discuss case narratives as an integral form of health disparities learning. The case narrative topics will include an interaction with a non-English speaking patient, an African American with concerns of trust within the health system, and difficulties with access to care as well as the barriers to viewing a patient as an individual.

A. Perzynski (✉)
Center for Health Care Research and Policy, The MetroHealth System,
Case Western Reserve University, Cleveland, OH, USA
e-mail: Adam.Perzynski@case.edu

I. Adebambo
Department of Family Medicine, The MetroHealth System, Cleveland, OH, USA

What Is the Session About?

We will present a health disparities case narrative which the audience will read for about 10 minutes. After this, we will use a structured discussion activity and have seminar participants describe how the narrative made them feel and what changes might be necessary to promote health for similar patients in the future. The activity will be opened to a maximum of 35 participants. Specific questions about the case presented will include discussion of racial concordance/discordance of healthcare providers, trust, and the potential for patient and provider biases to influence the quality of care as well as access to care. The seminar organizers will work with participants to identify the "core disparities" represented in the narrative and discuss evidence in the literature about this topic.

Why Is the Session Important?

Health disparities are present in the US population and affect health outcomes. Research conducted by the Joint Center for Political and Economic Studies indicated that direct medical expenditures could have been reduced by $229.4 billion from 2003 to 2006 by eliminating health disparities (LaVeist et al. 2009). Excess costs due to health disparities represent nearly one third of the total healthcare expenditures for racial and ethnic minorities (LaVeist et al. 2009). Health providers are in a position to affect positive change to reduce and/or eliminate this problem. It is important that we not only provide information and awareness but also be able to initiate reflective and critical thinking in the individual learner to create a change in attitude if needed. The use of case narratives is a potentially powerful and effective method for achieving this goal.

Objectives

1. After attending this session, participants will understand some of the issues that may cause health disparities.
2. Participants will understand the use of case narratives to engage and involve their learners in teasing out the complexities of healthcare system and individual issues that coalesce to create health disparities.

Suggested Timed Agenda

Introduce the case narrative—10 minutes
Break up into 4 small groups—5 minutes
Group structured discussion—30 minutes
Group feedback—10 minutes
Self-reflection and evaluation—5 minutes

Disparities Narratives Workshop Pre-post Evaluation Tool

Please circle the choice that best describes how much you agree or disagree with the following statements.

Question/Statement	Please circle your answer				
1. This class today held my interest in the subject matter.	Strongly disagree	Disagree	Neither disagree/agree	Agree	Strongly agree
2. I learned how some patients might feel the healthcare system is indifferent to their needs	Strongly disagree	Disagree	Neither disagree/agree	Agree	Strongly agree
3. Learning about health disparities taught me the important of patient narratives	Strongly disagree	Disagree	Neither disagree/agree	Agree	Strongly agree
4. This class should be required for all health professionals	Strongly disagree	Disagree	Neither disagree/agree	Agree	Strongly agree
5. The presentation of the narrative(s) was done well by the teacher(s)	Strongly disagree	Disagree	Neither disagree/agree	Agree	Strongly agree
6. The narrative(s) covered the topics in a new and interesting way	Strongly disagree	Disagree	Neither disagree/agree	Agree	Strongly agree
7. The narrative(s) helped me think about what patients might be going through	Strongly disagree	Disagree	Neither disagree/agree	Agree	Strongly agree
8. As a learner, I felt the objectives were well defined	Strongly disagree	Disagree	Neither disagree/agree	Agree	Strongly agree
9. The narrative(s) evoked strong feelings.	Strongly disagree	Disagree	Neither disagree/agree	Agree	Strongly agree
10. Health disparities occur more frequently than healthcare providers think about	Strongly disagree	Disagree	Neither disagree/agree	Agree	Strongly agree

References

LaVeist TA, Gaskin DJ, Richard P (2009) The Economic Burden of Health Inequalities in the United States. http://www.thomaslaveist.com/wp-content/downloads/Burden_Of_Health_Disparities_Final__Report.pdf

Discussion Guide for Health Disparities Case Narratives

Ifeolorunbode Adebambo, Adam Perzynski, and Sarah Shick

Narratives are a method of sharing information that has a special impact on the audience. A narrative personalizes the events of an individual's life experience to highlight barriers that some patients encounter when seeking care. The use of narratives is also very versatile. The depth and breadth of coverage can be extensive and is usually dependent on your learners and group. This means that some of these narratives can be discussed multiple times to fully explore all of the nuances. Narratives impart knowledge that often leads to a change in attitude. This chapter selects a few narratives as examples for facilitators to perform this deep dive and address multiple issues within a narrative.

While reading the narratives ask yourself the questions:

1. Is there a disparity going on in this case narrative?
2. What types of disparities may be involved?
3. How do you think the disparity directly affected this individual's care?

I. Adebambo
Department of Family Medicine, The MetroHealth System, Cleveland, OH, USA

A. Perzynski (✉)
Center for Health Care Research and Policy, The MetroHealth System, Case Western Reserve University, Cleveland, OH, USA
e-mail: Adam.Perzynski@case.edu

S. Shick
Department of Sociology, Case Western Reserve University, Center for Health Care Research and Policy, The MetroHealth System, Cleveland, OH, USA
e-mail: ses165@case.edu

© The Author(s) 2019
A. Perzynski et al. (eds.), *Health Disparities*,
https://doi.org/10.1007/978-3-030-12771-8_55

Questions and Discussion: Time to Leave by Bode Adebambo

Questions

1. What do the physician and patient have in common as women of color with mutual African heritage?
2. How are their stories and experiences different?
3. How might the differences in their background affect care?
4. How is this patient struggling to exert her own independence and sense of power in this situation?
5. How can you accommodate that as a provider?
6. Do you think her sister is right to be angry with her physician for not "making me [the patient] obey her"?
7. How should providers cope with situations like this when a patient chooses to reject potentially lifesaving treatment?
8. What ways can be used to accommodate this patient and provide the best care possible?
9. What other populations distrust the health-care system? How could you handle care of these populations?

Discussion

This story is an extreme case but not unique in that multiple real-world scenarios and challenges are outlined. These challenges include a health-care system that continues to focus on disease and pathology rather than the care of the whole person and a general failure to engage with and meet the needs of some of the most vulnerable patients. The health-care system continues to deliver care using a biomedical model focused on primarily on physical problems rather than incorporating other models that include the social determinants of health (Gehlert et al. 2008).

Over a decade of research has specifically highlighted the influence of trust on preventive health screenings for racial and ethnic minorities and minority women in particular (Halbert et al. 2006; O'Malley et al. 2004). Mistrust of the health-care system is based in history and an understanding of that history is necessary if we are to advance toward a more equitable health-care system. Black people have experienced disparities in care since the days of slavery when African Americans were bought and sold as the property of whites. While the Civil War ended with Robert Lee's surrender in 1865, it was not until 1970 that the longevity of black men caught up to that of white male Civil War veterans (Dine 2008). In discussions with her doctor, the patient in "Time to Leave" referred to a history of unethical governmental and medical experimentation on African Americans. This mistrust is likely at least partially based on knowledge of the historical facts of the 1932 Public Health Service, Tuskegee Study of Untreated Syphilis in the Negro Male (CDC 2008). Though the study was officially ended in 1972, the American Medical Association and the

Centers for Disease Control and Prevention (CDC) defended the continuation of this study in 1969, even though there was effective treatment available (CDC 2008).

"Time to Leave" also directs us to the inadequacies of our health-care environments in cultivating a comfortable and caring atmosphere for all patients regardless of their race, ethnicity, sexuality, or socioeconomic status. The electronic medical record provides comprehensive details on laboratory tests and diagnoses and is similarly capable of recording patient care preferences as well as psychological and social barriers to care. The psychosocial capabilities remain under-recognized and seldom used.

Efforts to reduce disparities have included programs to improve access, policies to increase workplace diversity, innovations to recruit and retain minority providers, implementation of accountable care organizations, and mandates for teaching of cultural competency. Cultural competence is an appropriate starting point in recognizing cultural differences across patient populations but according to Murray-Garcia strategies are necessary that promote a change in attitude through self-awareness and cultural humility. For example, community discussion panels involving health-care providers and community members can promote cross-cultural learning across racial, ethnic, and social status boundaries.

This narrative, though it is an extreme case, highlights the pervasive power that psychological and social conditions have on health. The social environment influences patient health-care decisions in ways that can be disastrous for individuals. However, we know that stories can impart knowledge and ultimately lead to a change in attitude.

A group of 35 students in graduate programs in nursing, public health, epidemiology, and biostatistics was asked to read the "Time to Leave" narrative and provide a written reflection. Below, we present some selected responses from the reflections which included anger, frustration, injustice, and sadness.

> I couldn't help but feel sorry for the woman and angry with her at the same time. I cannot imagine what it must feel like to completely mistrust the system, so much so that she would refuse screening, treatment and refused to deal with or listen to anyone who told her things she did not want to hear.

> There was a much deeper issue here than just a patient who didn't trust healthcare providers – she was deeply affected by many of the wrongdoings of the past and probably has valid reasons not to trust healthcare providers.

> Not only does disease kill people, but so does distrust and fear.

Questions and Discussion: How Can We Care for Everyone? By Christina Antenucci

Questions

1. Is health care a right or privilege?
2. How does one create community/family especially in times of need?
3. Could I have made her come to see me sooner?
4. Would things have been different if I had been part of her "community"?

5. Suggest ways in which the medical community can reach vulnerable populations.
6. What does the community of the future look like, and how can it respond to very real needs of our increasingly diverse population?

Discussion

Many people in our society believe in the concept of human rights and equality. The idea of social justice that supports all peoples includes believing in equal access to health care for all. A lack of this access to health care has been shown to affect the overall quality of care and health outcomes in our population. The United States is number 37 on the WHO 2017 list of world's health systems. One of the top goals for WHO is equity in health care.

Inequity in health care has been calculated to result in an increase in health-care expenditure projected by the Joint Center for Political and Economic Studies to be 229.4 billion during the years between 2003 and 2006. Thirty percent due to direct costs of health inequities and the rest indirect costs related to premature death and loss of work (LaVeist et al. 2009).

The Centers for Disease Control has used the maxim, "Health equity benefits everyone." every person who dies young, is avoidably disabled, or is unable to function at their optimal level represents not only a personal and family tragedy but also impoverishes our communities and our country. We are all deprived of the creativity, contributions, and participation that result from disparities in health status (Meyer et al. 2013).

Promoting healthy primary care relationships has been shown to improve health outcomes, but improvements to health-care interactions cannot address all barriers. Direct delivery of health care at best accounts for about 20% of an individual's health, and much of the rest are related to social determinants of health (Hood et al. 2016).

In this narrative, the clinician had a good relationship with her patient. Unfortunately, this was no match against her other challenges—poverty, race, sexual identity, age, and lack of family support. Studies have repeatedly shown that interventions directed only to health care are not adequate to deal with problems that affect a population (Thornton et al. 2016). Comprehensive targeted interventions are needed to see a decreased in disparities.

Questions and Discussion: Where Is the Patient? Finding the Person in Patient-Centered Health Care by Adam Perzynski, Carol Blixen & Martha Sajatovic

Questions

1. Has there been a time where you have seen the person instead of just a patient in front of you?
2. What are some of the reasons for depersonalization of patients in medicine?

3. How does depersonalization affect the accuracy of your patient histories, the maintenance of their chronic conditions, or the ability to monitor the patient's challenges to adherence of treatment recommendations?
4. How does this imbalance in power between the providers and patients play out in relation to the trust of health-care providers within certain vulnerable patient populations?
5. At the end of the narrative Mr. Green speaks of the providers finally finding him stating, "Do the providers and staff have a right to be angry?".
6. What are other ways that patients are expected to follow informal and formal rules in the health-care interaction? How do the rules and their enforcement vary for different patients such as a wealthy businessperson, a politician, a pastor, a single parent, a teenager, or a tattooed biker?
7. What are the diverse ways that race, age, socioeconomic status, gender, disability, and/or sexual orientation (or an intersection of such roles) influence these formal and informal rules?

Discussion

In the last decade, we have seen dramatic increases in US health-care costs which have been accompanied by less than dramatic increases in health-care quality, especially when compared to other developed nations. In addition, the US health-care system is characterized by persistent health disparities leading to premature mortality and unnecessary suffering for racial and ethnic minorities and persons of low socioeconomic status. Increasingly, policy discussions have focused on theories and processes that promote value-driven health care. Few disagree that health care should benefit patients, not do them harm, and should be accessible and affordable. Despite the strength of health-care transformation initiatives such as payment reform, health information exchange, the Patient Centered Medical Home and the Chronic Care Model, our health-care institutions seem unable to learn the lessons from simple failures in areas fundamental to promoting trust and confidence among people who receive health care.

Paramount among these failures is the loss of the person in processes that enhance the efficiency of the health-care system. The problems of "techno-medicine" have been described for many decades (Clarke et al. 2003), yet medicine is not alone in this regard. Technological advancements from the automobile and the assembly line to the mobile phone and internet shopping have altered the ways humans interact. Even the very pace at which technological change happens has accelerated, making it even more challenging to evaluate the influence of these changes on how people are treated as opposed to how many are treated or how many have reached one or another clinical threshold (Table 1).

Table 1 Some ways of defining persons who use health services

TIFKAP	Used frequently in the Netherlands, a derivative of "The Artist Formerly Known as Prince," but here "The Individuals Formerly Known as Patients" (Kremer et al. 2011).
Person	A being, such as a human, who has certain capacities or attributes constituting personhood. Personhood can be defined differently in different disciplines, cultures, times, and places.
Patient	Any recipient of health-care services. Etymological roots in Latin, "one who suffers."
Consumer	A person or group of people that are the final users of products and or services generated within a social system. The concept of a consumer may vary significantly by context.
Customer	The recipient of a good, service, product, or idea, obtained from a seller, vendor, or supplier for a monetary or other valuable consideration. A customer purchases goods, a consumer uses them.
Client	A person who receives help or advice from a professional person. Implies the role of consumer with decision-making authority. Implies a business transaction involving receipt of services.
Survivor	One who survives; one who endures through disaster or hardship. The concept of survivorship implies living in the context of difficult circumstances, but the actual circumstances might vary considerably.

Questions and Discussion: Testing Trust—Vivian Oluwatoyin Opelami

Questions

1. Does the same racial or ethnic heritage translate to the same experiences and histories?
2. Can this be an issue for people from different areas of the United States or different areas of the same city?
3. How can you work to accommodate these potential differences?
4. Consider social wounds that past generations have experienced such as the Tuskegee experiments or forced sterilizations of Puerto Rican women. What are some other examples of social wounds that have been suffer by Americans (immigrant or otherwise) that could affect patient trust in the provider, adherence to treatment, or even the patient's broader trust in society?
5. How can you work to build trust with a patient (or population) who has suffered such social wounds?
6. What are ways that a practice or hospital can adapt to help rebuild trust and provide better care?

Discussion

African Americans have clear reasons to mistrust the health-care system as per the narrative based on the knowledge of historical facts. In 1932, the Public Health Service, Tuskegee Study of Untreated Syphilis in the Negro Male is one such clear example (CDC 2008). Though the study was officially ended in 1972, the American Medical Association and the Centers for Disease Control and Prevention (CDC) defended the continuation of this study as late as 1969, even though there was effective treatment available (CDC 2008).

People often assumedly translate a shared ethnicity to mean similar shared experiences and sometimes make their choice of provider based on this assumption. In this narrative, although the provider and patient were of the same race, some of their experiences have been very different and others continue to be common. As the world becomes more diverse we should expect to see people of similar race or mixed race with different experiences. Honest communication with patients and an open, humble attitude shows cultural empathy (Murray-Garcia and Tervalon 1998). Such empathy can encourage the open exchange that occurred between this provider and patient. Such authenticity and openness served to improve the relationship between them and the quality of care.

There is some evidence that minority patients have improved care and satisfaction from providers of a similar race and ethnicity (DHHS-HRSA 2006). Trust in health care has been a difficult issue for minorities especially the African American population. There are not many studies that have looked directly at trust in the health-care system. Some indirect studies have looked at compliance for recommended health maintenance testing, another at the use of hospice facilities by minorities and another at the number of minorities that enroll in research studies. Results of the research enrollment study showed that if a person of similar race/ ethnicity asked the patients to enroll there was a larger number that enrolled. These results were similar with enrollment in hospice, with a higher number enrolling if it was presented by a heath care provider of similar ethnicity.

Questions and Discussion: The System Is Unfair—Wistler Saint-Vil

Questions

1. Is there bias in the treatment of pain based on race?
2. Should a race be excluded from a procedure in general because they "participate less"?
3. What are some reasons that disparities exist with kidney transplantation?
4. What recourse does his patient have if any?
5. What should your response be as a health-care provider?

Discussion

Health disparities in obtaining a kidney transplant as well as in the outcomes after a transplant continue to exist. The reasons are multiple and complex. There has been some progress made in recent years to address this disparity, but it is still far from equitable. The black donor education program funded by the National Center on Minority Health and Health disparities closed the gap relating to the ethnicity of donors by increasing the number of minority donors from 15% to 28.8% by 2001 (Callender et al. 2002). Despite this, the gap continued between the allocation and outcomes from kidney transplants.

In 2014, the United Network for Organ Sharing implemented a new kidney allocation system to reduce disparities among wait-listed patients. However, those in the position to make this change, such as dialysis clinic providers as well as the patients with ESRD, were unaware of how this policy change could improve access to kidney transplant (Harding et al. 2017).

Many other factors including genetics and racism have been highlighted in research and policymaking. The effect of racism manifests in several ways and has been classified as internalized, personally mediated, or institutionalized. Internalized racism is described as racism that occurs at the intrapersonal level. For example, African American patients might undervalue themselves and/or decide not to seek the best treatment available. Personally mediated racism occurs at the interpersonal level. For example, evidence suggests that some providers show unconscious racial bias that affects their treatment and care management decisions. Institutionalized racism can manifest at multiple levels such as institutions, community, and public policy. An example is the longstanding existence of racial residential segregation as well as known links between racial composition in the neighborhood and dialysis facility-level transplantation rates (Olufajo et al. 2017).

Multiple layers of disadvantage have contributed to disparities in outcomes for African American kidney transplant recipients. Data from analysis of the US transplant registry data, which included adult Caucasian or AA solitary kidney recipients undergoing transplantation between 1990 and 2009 comprising 202,085 transplantations, showed an estimated rate of 5-year graft loss decreased from 27.6% to 12.8% over 20 years. African Americans have a 10–20% poorer graft survival rate than all ethnic groups. This is true of living related donor transplants, unrelated donor or cadaver donor transplant. Thus, although the disparity for graft loss has significantly improved, equity is still far off, and other disparities, including living donation rates and delayed graft function rates, have widened during this time.

Questions and Discussion: The Irritable Uterus by Rebecca Fischbein, PhD

Questions

1. Is there a disparity in this narrative?
2. Can a challenging diagnosis be due to a disparity? Give examples.
3. What role does communication between patient and provider play in disparities?
4. How could you improve communication with this patient?

Discussion

Communication is an integral part of the patient/physician relationship, and multiple hours are spent teaching this skill through medical school and as ongoing education in practice. Better communication has been linked to patient compliance as well as fewer law suits against providers.

Clinical practice has shifted for many years to a patient centered model that encourages people to play an active role in their medical decision. Shared decision making requires a relationship between patient and provider that allows education and support. Research continues to demonstrate that the ability of a provider to communicate with a patient directly influences compliance with recommended treatment and clinical outcomes (AHRQ 2017).

Integral to communication is the willingness of the physician to educate and fully inform the patient of their medical condition and options (AHRQ 2017) such that they are able to make an informed decision. When practiced this has been shown to improve the quality of the decision, the communication as well as patient satisfaction. This is particularly important when providers are dealing with undifferentiated symptoms and signs.

Questions and Discussion: Barriers to the Breast by Sandra Esber

Questions

1. Discuss the limits of "educating" patients when their social and personal circumstances limit the application of that knowledge.
2. Are there times that you feel resentment toward a patient in such a scenario?

3. How can you show compassion and "get creative" with patients to adapt their care to their circumstances in life?
4. What assumptions have been made about this woman that may affect her care?
5. How would judgments have been different 50 years ago in a different racial climate and among different cultural norms about age of marriage, children, and number of children?

Discussion

Cleveland, Ohio is consistently ranked as one of the poorest large city in the United States with 54.4% of the children living in poverty (Exner 2014). Children are particularly vulnerable to disparities. According the Institute of Medicine, only 5% of studies on health-care disparities address disparities for children (Flores and Tomany-Korman 2008).

Breastfeeding is a health disparity that affects the health of both mother and child. Breastfeeding is associated with decreases in breast and ovarian cancers and quicker weight loss for the mother. For the child, overwhelming evidence shows decreases in obesity, diabetes, Sudden Infant Death Syndrome, asthma, allergies, and gastrointestinal problems (Eidelman et al. 2012). By not breastfeeding, a woman puts herself and her child at a higher risk for these problems.

Unfortunately, certain populations of mother's do not get the education and support that they need to make the decision to breastfeed. Moms who are successful with breastfeeding often have a family member who breastfed, have positive support for breastfeeding by family, friends, and especially the baby's father. Mothers that are ill-prepared to face the challenges that occur after they delivery with breastfeeding are more likely to give up breastfeeding.

Research shows that multiple contacts with health-care professionals and peer supports who educate moms on the benefits of breastfeeding at every prenatal visit can make a difference in a mom's expectation after delivery, her choice to breastfeed, and her ability to continue to breastfeed for the recommended minimum of six months (Renfrew et al. 2012).

Questions and Discussion: New in Town by John Boltri

Questions

1. What are her thoughts regarding her husband's diagnosis?
2. What role could her support system play?
3. How does one connect with a hurting patient?
4. How is communication related to years of education?

5. Should providers help their patient financially when they are able to do so?
6. How can this affect the patient-provider relationship?

Discussion

More than 1.5 million households and 3 million children in the United States get by on less than two dollars per day (Edin and Shaefer 2015). Many individuals and families have no regular source of income whatsoever and struggle to meet even the most basic of daily needs. The woman in the last narrative presented with mental health problems which directly affected her ability to take care of herself and ultimately her health. She managed to navigate her way to see a doctor and unfortunately had to be referred elsewhere to see a mental health specialist. Studies have shown that co-located mental health with primary care improves access and decreases the stigma associated with mental health (Kwan and Nease 2013). Integrated care environments can sometimes reduce fragmentation and streamline the process of meeting patient needs, heading off processes that lead to care disparities and circumventing some social constraints like transportation.

When her primary care doctor was able to arrange an appointment with a mental health specialist, the next barrier to overcome was transportation to get there. Patients frequently encounter situations where they do not have the money needed to receive care or treatment. There is little research evidence about providers giving gifts or money to patients to help with such expenses. Is there an acceptable amount to gift? What are the reasons to give money to patients? Who do we give to? Our behavior in giving monetary gifts is determined somewhat by the experience of nonprofit and charitable organizations.

Conventional wisdom might suggest that meeting needs rather than giving cash support directs the gift down a specific path determined by the giver rather than money which is directed by a recipient, thus potentially avoiding abuses. However, there is a strong counter argument which suggests that in many situations, for example in unfamiliar cultures, cash assistance may be more suitable. Recipients familiar with their own situation would know best how to maximize the results from having extra cash on hand. In this case not only did her improved appearance confirm the improvement in her mental health but she also returned the money.

Questions and Discussion: Rude by Bode Adebambo

Questions

1. Why did it take so long for the residents to realize the patient was blind?
2. How can we improve communication around disabilities?

3. What are the barriers to patients discussing personal disability?
4. Give examples of barriers to care that patients with different disabilities may encounter?
5. How can the health-care system and health-care providers break down some of these barriers?

Discussion

People with disabilities generally report poorer health than those without disabilities. Studies have shown that patients with disabilities are more likely to have problems with access. Some medical centers do not have ramps or appropriate equipment for access. The presence of pre-existing conditions also created challenges for disabled people in obtaining health insurance resulting in limited access to care. The Accountable Care Act and Medicaid expansion improved access to health care by removing that restriction but care is still far from equitable.

Recommended and required care for all such as health maintenance physicals are sometimes difficult as equipment needed such as weighing scales and proper examining tables are often not available precluding basic care. This resulted in women with mobility disorders less likely being up to date with their health maintenance such as mammograms and pap smears.

The data shows that the percentage of the population with disabilities increase with age. Some disabilities such as hearing, and vision are often not visible and can be easily missed. The absence of widespread teaching to health-care providers on the care of disabled patients acts as a barrier to patients receiving appropriate health care. Specific disabilities such as sensory loss have been shown to contribute to the incidence of delirium in hospitalized patients. Inquiring specifically about these disabilities in older people is extremely important as some patients who have lived with a disability for a long time have become accustomed to it. Being observant to nonverbal cues and increased sensitivity may yield greater benefit.

Questions and Discussion: Everyone Called Him Crazy by Veronica Cheung

Questions

1. Why do you think the patient thought his health-care providers were "racists"?
2. Do Asians in the United States experience racial and ethnic health disparities?
3. How do you think communication could have been improved with this patient?
4. How much time do you think should be spent with this patient during a visit?

Discussion

Asian Americans are a heterogeneous group with varying access to health care and health. Data from Department of HHS show that Asian American women have the highest life expectancy, 85.8 years, of any ethnic group in the United States (DHHS 2018). Among the subgroups highest are Chinese women, 86.1 years. Despite these numbers, disparities still exist in this population. The Asian American population are doing better than the index group in several factors including life expectancy and fewer heart disease; however, there continue to be disparities in several outcomes.

The leading cause of death in Asian Americans is cancer at 26.1% followed by heart disease at 22.8% in 2015. They have the highest prevalence of tuberculosis infection in the United States. The inability to speak English, just as the patient in the narrative, acts as a barrier to effective health care (DHHS 2018)

Questions and Discussion: The Struggles of the Undocumented by Chris Gillespie

Questions

1. How can neighborhood centers that cater to specific populations help to address and eliminate health disparities?
2. Next contrast the pros and cons of neighborhood centers and health disparities with the pros and cons of a large and very diverse community hospital or a less diverse small rural hospital.
3. How do you think trauma and stress can worsen or be worsened by health disparities?
4. How would you approach a patient in a compassionate way about the influence of trauma, stress, and health disparities on her/his health in a manner that is validating to the patient?

Discussion

The causes of health disparities are multiple and complex. Chronic stress in minority populations has been one of the causes suggested for the existence of disparities. This chronic stress related to ethnicity, and/or socioeconomic status contributes to the overall stress that minorities feel.

Some studies have shown a link between stress and chronic diseases such as heart disease, obesity, diabetes, and depression. Furthermore, ethnic groups that are already economically disadvantaged are even more susceptible to stresses related to low socioeconomic status (Warnecke et al. 2008). Community health centers are placed advantageously to interact with the community and explore their needs. A smaller health center is more adaptable in its ability to meet those needs. Any health center can create a bridge to community members by offering peer support to other patients going through similar experiences.

Questions and Discussion: The Fall that Keeps on Falling—Sarah Schick

Questions

1. Please comment on distrust within the health-care system and its impact on patients.
2. Does a patient's race affect how pain is treated?
3. What contributes to disparities among injured workers?
4. How does social support affect a patient's health?
5. What ways can a health-care provider improve the health of this group of patients (injured workers)?

Discussion

Several common themes arise in this and many other of my Workers' Compensation experiences—mutual distrust, both on my part and that of the system and care providers; stigma and discrimination; social support, both positive and negative; and an impact on my identity, self-esteem, and ability to fulfill social roles. In the moment, and even for several years afterward, I thought that what happened to me was unique. Yet, as I met other injured workers in waiting rooms and through volunteering as a peer counselor with an injured worker coalition, I learned that many of these elements were surprisingly common.

Compensation and coverage of care for injured workers has a long and complex history, with American Workers' Compensation laws enacted slowly state by state between the early to mid-1900 as a "no-fault" system that accepted workplace injuries as a natural occurrence in the labor market. Early resistance to adoption and implementation of laws, programs, and coverage arose from both employers and health-care professionals. Workers' Compensation was recognized as a way to protect employers from legal torts claims, and to distinguish coverage for permanent disability through Social Security. The Workers' Compensation system historically and currently offers injured workers protections through reimbursement for lost wages and medical care that is often otherwise cost-prohibitive due to lack of or limited health insurance coverage and high out-of-pocket expenses—though, in practice, the level of care and support actually received varies greatly (Guyton 1999).

On the surface, the mandated coverage of all workers through Workers' Compensation systems has the potential to minimize health disparities, yet structural factors put minorities and people from low socioeconomic backgrounds at higher risk for occupational injury. In addition, structurally driven barriers to care, including the adversarial and confrontational health-care interactions and lack of recognition or treatment of the complex biopsychosocial factors faced by injured workers compared to equivalent nonoccupational injuries, can increase disparities in access to treatment, care received, as well as worsen health outcomes and delay return to work (Chibnall et al. 2005; Scuderi et al. 2005; Krahn et al. 2015).

Lack of trust within health care, insurance, and other bureaucratic systems occurs frequently due to the inherent power imbalances and depersonalization that exist in such systems (Scuderi et al. 2005; Chibnall et al. 2005; Corroto 2011). Broader issues also come into play in the form of health disparities driven by stigma and subsequent discrimination based on race, ethnicity, gender, immigration status, sexual orientation, disability, and socioeconomic status that affect access to and quality of health care through conscious or subconscious bias on the part of providers, as well as through structural barriers in access to resources patients need to prevent or manage health issues (Krieger 2014; Phelan et al. 2010).

Minority patients tend to be more distrusting of their physicians, and physicians—particularly those treating patients for pain in clinics or emergency departments—can be significantly more distrusting of and less responsive to the needs of patients who are minorities, from low socioeconomic backgrounds, or receiving Workers' Compensation (Chibnall et al. 2005; Tamayo-Sarver et al. 2003). Mirroring health-care disparity trends in the broader population, African American injured workers receive significantly poorer quality of care and have worse outcomes than their Caucasian counterparts (Chibnall et al. 2005). Pain patients in general are treated with greater levels of skepticism by physicians, and, as with personal injury claims, injured workers are often suspected of catastrophizing and malingering for financial benefit (Scuderi et al. 2005; Tennyson 2008; Lipson and Doiron 2006).

While much of the literature about Workers' Compensation programs comes from a health-care or insurance perspective focuses on fraud, fraudulent mindsets, or negative patient behaviors, there is great variation in definitions of what constitutes fraud, in terms of both "hard" criminal fraud and the less clear "soft" fraud driven by abuse of the system or a disconnect between social norms of care and narrow bureaucratic limits on coverage prescribed by providers based on patient need (Tennyson 2008; Leigh 2011). Providers, claim reviewers, and researchers are habituated to assume fraud, often with assumptions that approximately 10% of claims are fraudulent, yet a detailed, nearly decade long review state and federal Workers' Compensation programs demonstrated that only 1–2% of cases were fraudulent (Tennyson 2008; Derrig and Zicko 2002, in Tennyson 2008).

Motivated by these assumptions, many injured workers are shadowed and tailed by fraud investigators videotaping their activities to "catch" them in some questionable activity, despite ample medical documentation and other types of evidence supporting the legitimacy of the claim, in order to prove the worker and treating physicians wrong or simply as a cost-saving practice for the system

(Lipson and Doiron 2006). Of course, there are some fraudulent Workers' Compensation claimants, but investigators surveil workers without consideration of the possibility that the worker may be dragging out a bag of trash or lifting up a crying child not out of an effort to scam the system or reject medical restrictions, but in desperation due to lack of support. Nor is the investigator likely to see, or record, the patient spending hours resting and recovering from pain caused lack of resources or supportive services that would prevent the perceived fraud in the first place.

While this mentality is popular on the evening news, it creates a highly fearful and disorienting environment for people who are already scared, in pain, feeling insecure, and have had their worlds upended completely. The contentious, adversarial approach focused on assumed negative worker behavior and personality traits appears in research, policy, and practice, and causes a vicious cycle where injured workers get worse because of the increased levels of stress, internalized stigma, lack of coverage for supportive/assistive services, and denial of care due to suspicion of fraud, which then creates physical and psychological symptoms worse than the original injury, in turn creating further suspicion of fraud, catastrophizing, or malingering (Pfau 2007; Lipson and Doiron 2006; Chibnall et al. 2005).

Examination of the burden of occupational injury and illness is challenging due to the fact that many injuries and illness are underreported, not approved when they should be, and there is inconsistent data collection across Workers' Compensation systems. However, estimates have shown that medical and nonmedical indirect costs are close to $200 billion dollars annually, with only a quarter of this financial burden carried by Workers' Compensation systems while the rest falls on injured workers, their families, and society to cover (Leigh 2011).

Injured workers face a process of denial or delay of prescribed treatments and medications that causes increased pain and impairment, numerous court visits to obtain approvals for treatment or have diagnoses added to their claim, fraud suspicions by secondary providers, independent medical examinations (by doctors paid specifically to refute the need for care), and prevalent fraud investigations. In the end, this creates significant financial costs and other burdens for the system, for well-intentioned health-care providers trying to advocate for and appropriately treat claimants, and especially for injured workers trying to heal and rebuild their lives (Scuderi et al. 2005; Lipson and Doiron 2006). These costs and burdens, including untreated severe pain, can cause so much strife that it drives some injured workers to suicide due to enormous financial, interpersonal, psychological, and physical strain (Kuo et al. 2012).

Consider the way that identity, the ability to fulfill roles, and the social network change an injured worker like myself, a spirited woman in her twenties who went to work as if it were any other day and, in an instant, due to an accident caused by owner negligence, found myself severely injured, confused, scared, in horrific pain, and facing a world where the people I thought were there to help me often treated me with suspicion and disregard. In the past I would take pride in a work project, run, hike, have a night out with friends, or write in a journal to express myself, have fun, or cope with stress. Like so many other injured workers, in an instant my entire life *and* my access to coping resources changed—I struggled to have the strength to take a shower or make food and needed hours-long naps to recover, and my limited energy was consumed by doctors' appointments, navigating a labyrinth of bureaucracy and managing often debilitating symptoms that varied by good days/bad days that proved to be difficult to consistently predict or prevent (Charmaz 1993). Many of the tasks that I once took for granted as part of my identity and independence were suddenly barely, if at all, possible.

For myself, or any person in this situation, one of the most crucial coping tools is social support for assistance in tasks that are no longer possible, financial assistance, and in terms of emotional support and efforts to rebuild self-esteem, identity, and social roles. Though there are variations based on factors including race, culture, and socioeconomic status, a person's social support network is recognized as a critically important resource for coping with major stressors in life, and can have profound impacts on well-being, health outcomes, and response to adversity based on the levels of anticipated vs. received support, sense of control, and the positive or negative appraisal of both stressors and social relationships (Pearlin et al. 2005; Kahana and Kahana 2018; Antonucci 2001).

People and interactions, who are a strain to the individual(s) undergoing a stressful situation, are likely to be appraised to as negative social relationships/support (e.g., difficult family or friends, an unaccommodating or discriminatory boss/coworkers, or an abusive partner who demands attention or care, regardless of circumstances). Though examples of negative social support may seem to be solely driven by malevolent actions or attitudes, they often arise from the individuals in a social network experiencing subconscious fear or stigma, ignorance about the illness/injury, feelings of helplessness, or general difficulty in coping with watching friend go through a stressful, traumatic event. For a person experiencing injury or illness, this actual or perceived negative social support can impact what is known as the "social scaffolding" or "convoy" of people around them and can lead to isolation, depression, decreased sense of control, and worse health outcomes (Rowlands 2001; Antonucci 2001).

Injured workers deal with complex physical, emotional, and bureaucratic issues, and social support is crucial in maintaining hope and the ability to heal. My boyfriend and my main Workers' Compensation physician (physician of record, or POR) are both strong examples of what I appraised to be positive sources of social support who offered trustworthiness, did not discriminate, and supported my efforts to rebuild my identity, self-esteem, and hope to fulfill my desired roles as a partner, mother, patient, and valued member of society. My boyfriend's presence in the emergency department, and in the multiple follow-up visits, was crucial for my emotional well-being, but also for keeping track of the vast amount of information that was being exchanged while I was in a weakened state.

My exchanges with my POR, strongly contrasted my interactions with the emergency department staff. At the time, he was a young physician starting his private occupational medicine practice, and was full of idealism and passion for advocacy that would never leave, but did tarnish slightly over a decade of battles with the Bureau of Workers' Compensation. The day I called my POR to tell him I was throwing up blood, he was concerned and kind, yet firm in his instructions to immediately proceed to the emergency department. He responded with elation upon learning about the pregnancy, but also offered a warning that it may affect my Workers' Compensation claim because they could not be sure which of my symptoms were coming from the injury and which arose from the strain of pregnancy, and would likely dismiss requests for treatment by blaming the latter. A few weeks later, when I called him to tell about the miscarriage, he did his best to sound as professional as usual but still choked up a bit, and was remarkably supportive in his comforting reassurance that I would rise above this challenge and perhaps one day even have another chance at motherhood.

In contrast, the flippant attitude of the triage nurse, the very matter of fact, detached attitude of the ED staff during the NG tube insertion, and the pervasive accusations of fraud were experienced by myself and my boyfriend as negative support, especially given our assumptions that we were in place meant to be a source of supportive care in a terrifying time. Another example of negative social support occurred while I was hospitalized for complications from the miscarriage. My boyfriend's best friend called to chastise him for not leaving the hospital to attend band practice and properly prioritize his commitment to them, since he'd already been spending a lot of time supporting me. This triggered additional strain, tension, and guilt for both of us during an already traumatic time in our lives.

The onset of an injury or illness, and the impact it has on an person's experiences, overall physical and mental health, and access to recourses needed to survive or thrive, can be a traumatic and life-changing event for anyone. Society in general, and health-care providers, policymakers, and institutions specifically, may be unaware of, underestimate, or intentionally overlook the many ways such a profoundly complex life-changing burden can influence overall well-being, health outcomes, financial resources, and participation in society. For injured workers, the compounded challenges arising from experiences of distrust and fraud suspicions, stigma and discrimination, changes in social support, and the negative impact on identity and ability to fulfill social roles creates additional burdens which take such an immense a toll that the initial injury becomes a vicious cycle of challenges—a fall that won't stop falling.

References

AHRQ (2017) 2016 National healthcare quality and disparities report. Agency for Healthcare Research and Quality, Rockville. AHRQ Pub. No. 17-0001. http://www.ahrq.gov/research/findings/nhqrdr/nhqdr16/index.html Accessed 31 Aug 2018

Antonucci TC (2001) Social relations an examination of social networks, social support. In: Birren JE, Schaie KW (eds) Handbook of the psychology of aging, vol 3, 5th edn. Academic Press, New York, p 427

Callender CO, Miles PV, Hall MB, Gordon S (2002) Blacks and whites and kidney transplantation: a disparity! but why and why won't it go away? Transplant Rev 16(3):163–176

Centers for Disease Control (2008) U.S. public health service syphilis study at Tuskegee. Available: http://www.cdc.gov/tuskegee/timeline.htm. Accessed 31 Aug 2018

Charmaz K (1993) Good days, bad days: the self in chronic illness and time. Rutgers University Press, New Brunswick

Chibnall JT, Tait RC, Andresen EM, Hadler NM (2005) Race and socioeconomic differences in post-settlement outcomes for African American and Caucasian Workers' Compensation claimants with low back injuries. Pain 114(3):462–472

Clarke AE, Shim JK, Mamo L, Fosket JR, Fishman JR (2003) Biomedicalization: technoscientific transformations of health, illness, and US biomedicine. Am Sociol Rev 1:161–194

Corroto C (2011) A postmodern headache. Qual Inq 17(9):854–863

Department of Health and Human Services Office of Minority Health (2018) Asian American profile. https://minorityhealth.hhs.gov/omh/browse.aspx?lvl=3&lvlid=63. Accessed 1 Sept 2018

Derrig RA, Zicko V (2002) Prosecuting insurance fraud—A case study of the massachusetts experience in the 1990s. Risk Manage Insur Rev 5(2):77–104

Dine SB (2008) Wartime health disparities and their aftermath. Health Affairs 27(4):1191

Edin K, Shaefer HL (2015) Two dollars a day: living on almost nothing in America. Houghton Mifflin Harcourt, New York

Eidelman AI, Schanler RJ, Johnston M, Landers S, Noble L, Szucs K, Viehmann L (2012) Breastfeeding and the use of human milk. Pediatrics 129(3):e827–e841

Exner R (2014) Decade after being declared nation's poorest big city, 1-in-3 Clevelanders remain in poverty. http://www.cleveland.com/datacentral/index.ssf/2014/09/decade_after_being_declared_na.html. Accessed 31 Aug 2018

Flores G, Tomany-Korman SC (2008) Racial and ethnic disparities in medical and dental health, access to care, and use of services in US children. Pediatrics 121(2):e286–e298

Gehlert S, Sohmer D, Sacks T, Mininger C, McClintock M, Olopade O (2008) Targeting health disparities: a model linking upstream determinants to downstream interventions. Health Affairs 27:339–349

Guyton GP (1999) A brief history of workers' compensation. Iowa Orthop J 19:106

Halbert CH, Armstrong K, Gandy OH Jr, Shaker L (2006) Racial differences in trust in health care providers. Arch Intern Med 166:896

Harding K, Mersha TB, Pham PT, Waterman AD, Webb FJ, Vassalotti JA, Nicholas SB (2017) Health disparities in kidney transplantation for African Americans. Am J Nephrol 46(2):165–175

Hood CM, Gennuso KP, Swain GR, Catlin BB (2016) County health rankings: relationships between determinant factors and health outcomes. Am J Prev Med 50:129–135

Kahana E, Kahana B (2018) Contextualizing successful aging: new directions in an age-old search. In Lives in Time and Place and Invitation to the Life Course (pp. 225–255). Routledge

Krahn GL, Walker DK, Correa-De-Araujo R (2015) Persons with disabilities as an unrecognized health disparity population. Am J Public Health 105(S2):S198–S206

Kremer JA, Van Der Eijk M, Aarts JW, Bloem BR (2011) The individual formerly known as patient, TIFKAP. Miner Med 102(6):505

Krieger N (2014) Discrimination and health inequities. Int J Health Serv 44(4):643–710

Kuo CJ, Gunnell D, Chen CC, Yip PS, Chen YY (2012) Suicide and non-suicide mortality after self-harm in Taipei City, Taiwan Br J Psychiatry 200(5):405–411

Kwan BM, Nease DE (2013) The state of the evidence for integrated behavioral health in primary care. In: Integrated behavioral health in primary care. Springer, New York, pp 65–98

LaVeist TA, Gaskin DJ, Richard P (2009) The economic burden of health inequalities in the United States. Joint Center for Political and Economic Studies, Washington, DC. Available at http://www.jointcenter.org

Leigh JP (2011) Economic burden of occupational injury and illness in the United States. Milbank Q 89(4):728–772

Lipson JG, Doiron N (2006) Environmental issues and work: women with multiple chemical sensitivities. Health Care W Int 27(7):571–584

Meyer PA, Yoon PW, Kaufmann RB (2013) Introduction: CDC health disparities and inequalities report-United States. MMWR Suppl 62(3):3–5

Murray-Garcia J, Tervalon M (1998) Cultural humility versus cultural competence: a critical distinction in defining physician training outcomes in multicultural education. J Health Care Poor Underserved 9:117–125

Olufajo OA, Adler JT, Yeh H, Zeliadt SB, Hernandez RA, Tullius SG, Backhus L, Salim A (2017) Disparities in kidney transplantation across the United States: does residential segregation play a role? Am J Surg 213(4):656–661

O'Malley AS, Sheppard VB, Schwartz M, Mandelblatt J (2004) The role of trust in use of preventive services among low-income African-American women. Prev Med 38:777–785

Pearlin LI, Schieman S, Fazio EM, Meersman SC (2005) Stress, health, and the life course: some conceptual perspectives. J Health Soc Behav 46(2):205–219

Pfau H (2007) To know me now. Qual Soc Work 6(4):397–410

Phelan JC, Link BG, Tehranifar P (2010) Social conditions as fundamental causes of health inequalities: theory, evidence, and policy implications. J Health Soc Behav 51(1_suppl):S28–S40

Renfrew MJ, McCormick FM, Wade A, Quinn B, Dowswell T (2012) Support for healthy breastfeeding mothers with healthy term babies. Cochrane Database Syst Rev 5:CD001141

Rowlands A (2001) Breaking my head in the prime of my life: acquired disability in young adulthood. In: Priestley M (ed) Disability and the life course: global perspectives, Cambridge University Press, Cambridge, UK/ New York, p 179

Scuderi GJ, Sherman AL, Brusovanik GV, Pahl MA, Vaccaro AR (2005) Symptomatic cervical disc herniation following a motor vehicle collision: return to work comparative study of workers' compensation versus personal injury insurance status. Spine J 5(6):639–644

Tamayo-Sarver JH, Hinze SW, Cydulka RK, Baker DW (2003) Racial and ethnic disparities in emergency department analgesic prescription. Am J Public Health 93(12):2067–2073

Tennyson S (2008) Moral, social, and economic dimensions of insurance claims fraud. Soc Res 75(4):1181–1204

Thornton RL, Glover CM, Cené CW, Glik DC, Henderson JA, Williams DR (2016) Evaluating strategies for reducing health disparities by addressing the social determinants of health. Health Affairs 35(8):1416–1423

US Department of Health and Human Services (2006) The rationale for diversity in the health professions: a review of the evidence. Health Resources and Services Administration, Bureau of Health Professions, https://www.hrsa.gov/advisorycommittees/bhpradvisory/cogme/Publications/diversityresourcepaper.pdf. Accessed 1 Sept 2018

Warnecke RB, Oh A, Breen N, Gehlert S, Paskett E, Tucker KL, Lurie N, Rebbeck T, Goodwin J, Flack J, Srinivasan S (2008) Approaching health disparities from a population perspective: the National Institutes of Health Centers for Population Health and Health Disparities. Am J Public Health 98(9):1608–1615

Review of Community Health Needs Assessment for Increasing Awareness and Reducing Disparities

Aleece Caron, Joseph Jaeger, Miriam Bar-on, and Kathryn Andolsek

Overview

Healthcare disparities/inequities have been identified as a critical aspect of health-care quality, and included as part of the Accreditation Council for Graduate Medical Education (ACGME) Clinical Learning Environment Review (CLER). As one would expect, addressing healthcare disparities is a universal challenge requiring the collaboration of graduate medical education (GME) educators and leaders. There are many opportunities to develop learning activities and assessment strategies in approaching healthcare disparities for our learners, faculty, and patients.

The purpose of this workshop is to bring together GME educators, healthcare system leaders, and other learners to share strategies and promote engagement in clinical site initiatives that act to address healthcare disparities. The session begins with a short presentation about health disparities, care inequities, and social determinants to set the stage. Through a mini-didactic and a hands-on experience, participants are then introduced to the Community Health Needs Assessment (CHNA). A CHNA and an implementation plan to address identified needs are required every 3 years of tax-exempt hospitals as a result of the Patient Protection and Affordable Care Act. Using the criteria for performing a CHNA, small groups will identify the required components through a "scavenger hunt" in an assigned document.

A. Caron (✉)
The MetroHealth System, Cleveland, OH, USA
e-mail: acaron@metrohealth.org

J. Jaeger
Monmouth Medical Center, Long Branch, NJ, USA

M. Bar-on
University of Nevada, Las Vegas, Las Vegas, NV, USA

K. Andolsek
Duke University, Durham, NC, USA

© The Author(s) 2019
A. Perzynski et al. (eds.), *Health Disparities*,
https://doi.org/10.1007/978-3-030-12771-8_56

Facilitators can find these documents easily which are publicly available on the websites of all tax-exempt hospitals and many other healthcare institutions. Facilitators hold a brief discussion focused on how they addressed the expectations outlined in the CLER Pathways to excellence document. Participants will then return to their small groups to select a specific content area identified in their CHNA and apply the CLER pathways properties to develop an educational experience or other quality initiative at their institutions. In doing so, both educational and administrative components of implementation are actively addressed. Participants should be further encouraged to highlight potential community and organizational partners or other available community resources that exist outside the walls of the healthcare system. The session ends with group report outs and a general debriefing to share feedback and identify potential next steps.

Pre-work (Optional but Encouraged)

1. Participants are sent an electronic link to Project Implicit, and encouraged to take an implicit association test (https://implicit.harvard.edu/implicit/takeatest.html).
2. Participants are sent a Community Health Needs Assessment and asked to review it.
3. Participants are asked to locate their own institution's or a peer institution's CHNA, review it and bring to the session.

Timed Session Agenda

1. Mini-didactic—disparities and CHNA 15 minutes
2. Small group work—scavenger hunt with assigned CHNA (attendees will be seated by CHNA received) 15 minutes
3. Small group work—design of educational activity 25 minutes
4. Large group volunteer report out of educational activity and discussion 15 minutes

Participation Guidelines

1. Two small group sessions during which participants will be asked to interact with members of the group

   (a) Small group session 1: scavenger hunt—a template of items needed to be identified within the assigned CHNA; participants will be seated by the

CHNA received in order to search together for the items requested. They will have been asked to review the CHNA prior to the session.

(b) Small group session 2: educational activity design—each small group will be challenged to develop at least one educational activity organized using a template

2. Large group report out and discussion—participants will have the opportunity to present their educational activity and discuss both the educational opportunities and the administrative challenges moving their activity forward.

Template Workshop Handout

DATE _____
List the names and emails of the members of your table

Name	Email
_____	_____
_____	_____
_____	_____
_____	_____
_____	_____

1. Identify three or more disparity(ies)/inequity(ies) by reviewing the part of the CHNA you have been given. How would you prioritize them?

2. Describe how a CHNA can be used with learners to address healthcare disparities/inequities.

3. Design an educational initiative for a group of learners (e.g. students, residents, fellows, or faculty (using the template on the next page) from one of the disparities/inequities identified in the CHNA.

Who are your Learners (check all that apply)		What is the anticipated level of learning activity (per Dreyfus model)?	
Residents/fellows		Novice	
Med students		Advanced Beginner	
PA/NP students		Competent	
Faculty		Proficient	
Other (list)		Expert	

Disparity/Inequity
identified:_____

Analyze the reason(s) for the disparity(ies)inequity(ies).

Identify the team: List the types/characteristics of individuals who could help with the
development and implementation of this activity.

List the Learning objectives for the initiative:

Describe the Learning plan and activities to address the disparity/inequity.

List needed/potential resources.

Outcome measures:
    a. Describe how you will measure the impact of the initiative on your learners and what
       specifically they have learned.

    b. Describe how you will measure the impact of the educational initiative on the
       disparity/inequity itself.

References

AAMC Analysis in Brief. https://www.aamc.org/download/419276/data/dec2014community-
    health.pdf. Accessed 1 Sept 2018
AAMC Toolkit: Communities, Social Justice and Academic Medical Centers. https://www.aamc.
    org/initiatives/research/healthequity/. Accessed 1 Sept 2018
Centers for Disease Control 2015 CDC Community Health Improvement Navigator. http://www.
    cdc.gov/chinav/. Accessed 1 Sept 2018
Michener JL, Koo D, Castrucci BC, Sprague JB (eds) (2015) The practical playbook: public health
    and primary care together. Oxford University Press, New York
Van Schaik E, Howson A, Sabin J (2014) Healthcare disparities. MedEdPORTAL 10:9675. https://
    doi.org/10.15766/mep_2374-8265.9675. Accessed 1 Sept 2018

Intersectionality Game

Sarah Shick

Intersectionality goes hand in hand with learning about health disparities. Each social or physical category that may create a disparity does not exist in a vacuum. One cannot separate the trans, the woman, the African-American, the poverty, or the disability. Each trait influences the other not in an additive way but in a multiplicative sense.

What does that mean? Imagine being asked to carry a series of bags, and the first bag weighs five pounds. Perhaps one might expect the second bag to weigh the same amount, so that the total load would be ten pounds. Instead, the burden carried multiplies and you're stuck with twenty-five pounds. Being a woman may be the equivalent to a five-pound bag in our society, but being an African-American woman would be a 25-pound bag, and being a disabled, trans, African-American woman would be a 625-pound bag to carry because of the way our society compounds theses social states into a significant burden.

This example is extremely simplistic, because each weight is not equal. Consider how the stigma and any social judgment vary by each category, limiting opportunities which can negatively influence overall health and social, economic, and educational opportunities. Here's a game to help you understand how arbitrary and difficult these social states can be and how the intersectionality of these states can drastically change one's experience in life.

Step 1: Have people pull five pieces of paper from five different hats or bags (one from each), with each hat containing a different color of writing on it (purple, green, red, black, and gold ink). On each piece of paper will be numbers (0, 5, 10, 50, 75, 100)—there can be extra sheets left over in the hats/bags. Once everyone has drawn their papers, have them total their scores.

S. Shick (✉)
Department of Sociology, Case Western Reserve University, Center for Health Care Research and Policy, The MetroHealth System, Cleveland, OH, USA
e-mail: ses165@case.edu

© The Author(s) 2019
A. Perzynski et al. (eds.), *Health Disparities*,
https://doi.org/10.1007/978-3-030-12771-8_57

209

Step 2: Once the scores are totaled, we'll give them the "cost" of certain things and instruct them to think about what is most important/desirable to them:

- Purchasing a home—100
- Advanced degree—50
- Children—50 each child
- Comprehensive health care—25 for individual, 75 for family
- Traveling—50
- Sustainable income from good job—50

Step 3: At this point the students will have scores between 500 and 25 and will be thinking about these scores as being bonuses and what they may "buy" with them. Time to flip the script. State to all of the students that when they were "born" they all started with 500 points, but these pieces of paper represent different socially constructed barriers in their lives.

- If they have a purple one, that is health, and a 0 is perfect health, but if it is a 100, it means they are severely disabled—so take that away from their original 500 points.
- Green is race, so if you got a score of 0 you are white, whereas a score of 100 is a recent immigrant.
- Red is gender, so that 0 is male, 50 is female, 75 is non-binary, and 100 is trans.
- Black is SES, so that 0 is extremely wealthy/privileged and 100 is abject poverty/homelessness.
- Random chance is gold and it is only eight marked papers (two each of: "add 50," "add 100," "subtract 50," "subtract 100") in with a bunch of blank papers.

Each score is subtracted from the 500 to give students an idea of how socially constructed concepts detract from their life chances. Then explain that a different society (or different time in the same society) could change that, e.g., if you were an Irish immigrant in the early 1900s, then that would count the same as a Central American immigrant does today, but now Irish immigrant status puts someone as a 0 in the race category.

Discussion Questions—How does that make you feel? How does it feel to think that you're winning with numbers, or have these chances, only to realize that a randomly selected number with an arbitrarily assigned value limited the possibilities you have for your life? How did you adjust your choices/goals from #2 in order to accommodate for the new math? How did that affect your choices and your motivation? How would this play out in a different country or at a different point in history?

Sensitization as the First Step: The Horatio Alger Exercise

Varun U. Shetty and S. Jeffrey Mostade

A deep awareness of privilege and oppression is necessary for one to be empathetic toward those less privileged. Before one even begins to grasp the concepts of privilege and oppression, one needs to be sensitized to one's own place in society and unearned privilege. This exercise is meant to be the beginning of a discussion, not an end. It seeks to sensitize participants to the existing disparities that are a result of unearned privilege. Unearned privileges involve being born into a system of oppression that devalues one race or culture over another, certain classes over others. Once one is sensitized, the educator can then move on to delve in deeper discussions of unearned privilege and disparity (Shetty and Magliola 2016).

Relating Experience to Health and Medical Education

Health and medical professions have a long history of training students to be emotionally detached from patients, and objectively assess patients' physical and mental symptoms (Halpern 2003). Although patients seek empathy from their physicians, the effectiveness of experiencing clinical empathy and compassion has been a contested area of medical training in the United States since at least the 1950s (Halpern 2003). It has been argued that empathy, for physicians, should rather be defined as detached objectivity (Halpern 2003, p. 670). Research has shown that physicians who incorporate an understanding of their patient's psychosocial dimensions into their patient interactions communicate better with those patients. Further, physicians can be taught these skills (Levinson 1995). There are physician barriers to the experience of empathy that can interfere with learning to use it as a tool in

V. U. Shetty (✉)
Internal Medicine-Pediatrics, The MetroHealth System, Cleveland, OH, USA

S. J. Mostade
Shaker Heights, OH, USA

© The Author(s) 2019   211
A. Perzynski et al. (eds.), *Health Disparities*,
https://doi.org/10.1007/978-3-030-12771-8_58

communication. Three of the barriers include anxiety (such as that introduced by the time pressure of the clinical interview), physicians negating psychosocial aspects of the patient as an important part of the illness or the cure, and finally, the negative emotions experienced by physicians occasionally with some patients (Halpern 2003).

The Horatio Alger exercise allows physicians and health practitioners to understand the complexities of privilege in society through personal experience of feelings and the processing of those feelings, therefore empathizing with others at an emotional rather than purely intellectual level. The importance of this initial experiential understanding of the inherent unfairness of society cannot be overemphasized, especially with health professionals who deal with the consequences of disparity and inequity every day. The versatility of this exercise lends itself to be adapted in different situations, specifically in global health, where unearned privilege, health-care disparities, and inequities are all magnified. This exercise can serve as an important tool to discuss and teach medical and allied health sciences students the various concepts of social justice and far-reaching health effects of an unequal society.

Background

Horatio Alger Jr. was a nineteenth century American author whose stories had a common theme of a poor, hardworking person rescued from their condition usually with an extraordinary act of bravery, determination, or honesty. This may have led to the common and often inaccurate presumption in the United States that anyone can escape his or her condition with hard work and determination. It is often forgotten that unequal employment and educational opportunities and health disparities are built into our socioeconomic system. The US economic condition is such that social mobility has declined since the 1980s, that is, a person is destined to remain near the economic position into which one was born (Semuels 2016). The Horatio Alger exercise was originally developed to expose the racial prejudices and unearned privilege that influenced a variety of situations in US life. We believe that this exercise can also be used to evoke empathy and understanding of health-care disparities that come with inequities in access to health care in the United States, but also in global health settings.

Unlearning Oppression workshops facilitated by Dr. Beth Blue Swadener and Dr. Mary Smith Arnold of Kent State University in 1995 included versions of the Horatio Alger exercise. This anti-oppression work was an extension of the Iowa City Women Against Racism Committee and the Women's Resource & Action Center from the 1980s through the 1990s (Grant 1999). It is often used a sensitization exercise for graduate students in counseling, social work, and other social services fields and is used as a perspective-taking exercise to form an emotional basis for accurate empathy (the client knows that they have been understood) (Connor 1994).

Objectives

The primary objective is to illustrate unearned privilege, oppression, disparity within an audience where it is not always apparent. This exercise aims to use the Horatio Alger exercise to expose, first the inequities built into our society, and then use that to understand health-care disparities inherent to the world we live in. Accurate empathy allows the patient to feel understood; if accurate empathy is the goal, it can be learned. Arbeitman proposed four components to the development of empathy: "affective sensitivity (experiencing the experience of the other), role-taking (acts of imagination), emotional responsiveness and empathic communication"(Connor 1994). This exercise provides the opportunity to experience affective sensitivity, role taking, and emotional responsiveness. A skilled facilitator can help the participants relate this directly to their practice with patients and students in a local or global setting.

The Exercise

The Horatio Alger exercise involves having people line up horizontally in a room and then move a step forward or backward depending if the sentence spoken applies to them. An alternate form of the exercise can be used if the space is quite large and the participants many. Participants can step toward the center and away, processing their relative positions at the reflection stage of the exercise. The authors have been very comfortable with the linear position arrangement as the relative positions are quite clear by the end of the exercise. Figure 1 shows a group of medical residents at the beginning of the exercise, and Fig. 2 shows the same group at the end of the exercise. The sentences that form part of the exercise demonstrate presence or absence of unearned privilege. At the end of the exercise, the person with most privilege ends up in the front of the room and one with the least, in the back. The exercise therefore brings to the physical realm, a concept that is largely abstract. It can sometimes make people uncomfortable, especially if one has not processed these ideas before.

Requirements

1. Time: 45–90 minutes. Preferably 90 minutes, especially if a larger group.
2. Space: Room large enough to accommodate participants, with lots of room lengthwise to allow for demonstration of difference between people in the front of the line and people in the back.

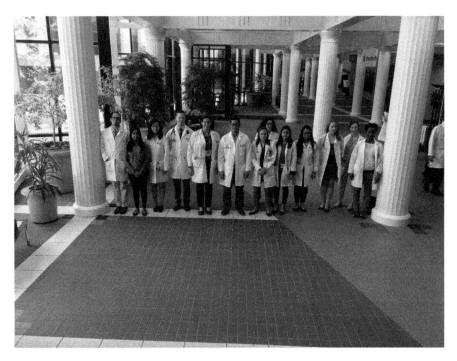

Fig. 1 Medicine-pediatrics residents beginning the Horatio Alger exercise

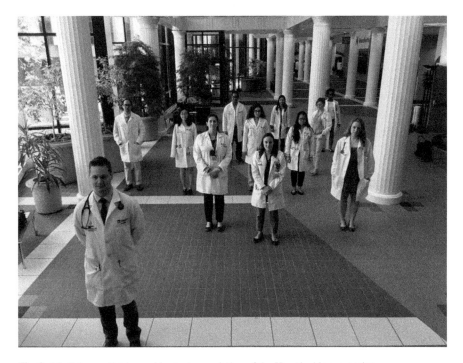

Fig. 2 Medicine-pediatrics residents at completion of the Horatio Alger exercise

Method

Set the Stage

Facilitate participants becoming comfortable with each other. This might be easier to do if your audience is made of residents, nurses, or allied health professionals who have been with each other for more than a year. You could ask them to pair up and come up with reasons why they came to this workshop, or what they think they would gain out of this workshop. If participants are completely new to one another, then propose a professional interview about their training. Avoid people from joining in late. It will cause confusion and will dilute the effect of the exercise.

Explain the Exercise

Make it clear that this exercise will require participant cooperation, willingness to be open, and intention not to possibly fear to feel strong emotions in the presence of so many others, because others will likely have similar feelings. Likewise, asking for relative confidentiality will not ensure, but assure, participants of the earnestness of co-participants.

Conduct the Exercise

Ensure that there is enough room to move in the space provided. Room setup will depend on the number of expected participants and the room arrangement, if there are desks, permanent fixtures, etc. The easiest setup is often accomplished in conference rooms with easily moveable chairs. Try to envision the number of expected participants moving across the room and allow for at least 20 forward steps, or the same number of question/prompts that you will provide to your group. Refrain from moving chairs, desks, etc. right before the exercise as this might dilute the effect of the exercise. Prepare the room beforehand.

When reading the statements, consider reading the statements in the order of least sensitive to most sensitive. This may increase the chances of honest responses amongst the delegates. This was suggested in the study conducted by the authors in which the general level of reported honesty was very high (Shetty et al. 2017).

Process People's Thoughts and Feelings

Personally experiencing privilege and oppression can often be difficult, revealing, and embarrassing. Participants often stand in the position of both oppressed and privileged at the same time – consider a person of color at a medical school or a person of European descent who is differently abled. Shape the experience of participants by asking questions but also reminding them that no amount of hard work or merit can change where they start the exercise. Remind them that no matter the feelings of guilt or fault that a participant may experience, that all the starting positions were brought about the circumstances of birth, and not by choice. Much of unearned privilege is multigenerational and hard to experience on any portion of the continuum. Help your participants to talk about experiences of multiple oppressions or intersectionalities, e.g., a lesbian, woman of color (Yeung and Pliner 2016).

Strong feelings can emerge and one needs to be sensitive and careful. Ask if anyone would like to reflect on being in their position, either front, middle, or back of the room. If nobody volunteers, consider picking on the person in the front first. Ask them how they feel about being in the front. Surprised? Indignant? Disbelief? Some might get angry, refusing to accept the position of relative privilege. Some, in the back, may be sad, ashamed, embarrassed. Be sure to consider these possibilities, and try to make them comfortable to see the differences, the disparities that are inherent in the society, but not visible. That is exactly the point of the exercise.

Know Your Audience

It can be helpful to tailor your questions according to the kind of audience you have. For example, if you seemingly have only European-American people, focus on gender and class issues; if only males, focus on race, ethnic, and class issues; if it's an audience in India, then tailor questions on caste, class, and gender grounds. There is disparity everywhere, the facilitator works to help the group understand their diversity and any unearned privilege.

Approach Every Comment with a Sense of Curiosity: Processing Tough Conversations

There will be many instances when participants will be uncomfortable after the exercise. You might be faced with anger or outright rejection of the validity of the exercise. It is important to not get deterred by such comments, and remember that this is simply people's discomfort being expressed in different ways. It is important to approach such comments with a sense of curiosity. "What would you like others to understand?" "What about your personal experience informs your opinion?", "Does anyone else in the room have some feelings or thoughts about this?" or simply, "Tell me more about that". One will see that every comment or opinion will lead to a deeper discussion about what it means to be in that relative position of privilege in the room. Help them remember that none of the unearned privilege involved merit, but simply the circumstances of birth. Talk about how this understanding may affect their understanding or communication with patient.

Tension sometimes experienced as a result of this anti-oppression work has been theorized to be a result of the hidden context and meanings ascribed by people to various cultural, racial, or other identities of experiential disparity. These oft-hidden meanings emerge during discussion of unearned privilege and access (Sue 2015). Five strategies for successfully facilitating tough discussions concerning racial and cultural diversity are offered by D.W. Sue, a professor of counseling psychology and researcher of cultural diversity. The workshop faculty should understand their racial/cultural identity; acknowledge and be open to admitting personal racial biases; validate and facilitate discussion of feelings; control the process, not the content, of race talk; and validate, encourage, and express admiration and appreciation to participants who speak when it feels unsafe to do so (Sue 2015).

Making It Your Own

The Horatio Alger exercise lends itself to modification quite easily. The statements must demonstrate unearned privilege. Earned privilege must not be included in the statements. Ensure that the statements are accurate statistically and are devoid of any ambiguity in meaning. If using a global health perspective for a western audience, you can evoke disparities and process the questions before bringing up the global health focused questions. These could highlight the common privilege that we all have here in developed economies. In another instance, if one is conducting the exercise in India, one may want to modify the questions that include caste and social class much more than race as in the Indian society, caste and class disparities are far more common than racial disparities. You can make any number of statements based on real statistics and apply it to your audience. When picked correctly, the effect can be poignant.

Statements

1. Insurance coverage for black, Hispanic, and Native American populations is significantly lower compared with White, non-Hispanic, and Asians. Take a step back if you are black, Native American, or Hispanic.
2. All those who went to a private school before college, take one step forward.
3. All those who were raised in a community where the vast majority of the police, politicians, and government workers were not of their ethnic or racial group, take one step back.
4. All those who commonly see people of their race or ethnicity as heroes or heroines on TV programs or movies, take one set forward.
5. All those who commonly see people of their race or ethnicity as heroes or heroines on TV programs or movies in roles you consider degrading, take one step backward.

6. All those whose ancestors were slaves in the United States, take one step back.
7. All those whose parents spoke English as a first language, take one step forward.
8. All those who have vacationed in a foreign country before their 18th birthday, take one step forward.
9. All those who had to take loans for college/medical school, take one step back.
10. All those who've been taken to art galleries or museums by their parents, take one step forward.
11. All those who have an immediate family member who is a doctor or lawyer, take one step forward.
12. All those who were educated in schools where the vast majority of the faculty members and staff were of your racial or ethnic group, take one step forward.
13. Non-elderly Hispanics have the highest uninsured rate, with nearly one in three lacking coverage (32%), followed by American Indians/Alaska Natives (27%), Blacks (21%), and Asians/Pacific Islanders (18%), who are all more likely than Whites (13%). All blacks, Native Americans, and Hispanics, take one step back (KFF.org).
14. Even though the majority of Hispanics, Blacks, and American Indians/Alaska Natives have at least one full-time worker in the family, they are more than twice as likely to be poor than Whites (KFF.org). Hispanics, Blacks, and Native Americans, take one step back.
15. If you had negative role models of your identity (religious affiliation, gender, sexual orientation, class, ethnicity) when you were growing up, take one step back.
16. If you can turn on the television or open the front page of the paper and see people of your ethnicity or sexual orientation widely represented, take one step forward.
17. Infant mortality rate is highest for non-Hispanic blacks and Native Americans. Non-Hispanic blacks and Native Americans, take one step back.
18. Hispanic women have the lowest percentage of primary care doctors in the United States. Hispanic women, take one step back (KFF.org).
19. If, as a child, you had a room of your own with a door, move one step forward.
20. If you have spent 1 year or more without health insurance, take one step backward.
21. If you've never had to hand a grocery store cashier food stamps for your food, move forward.
22. If you were rewarded as a child for being assertive and speaking your mind, move forward.
23. If most medical models for disease are based on your racial group, move forward.
24. If one or both of your parents never completed high school, move one step back.
25. If you can easily find birthday/valentine's day cards picturing people of your skin color, move one step forward.

26. If your bags have never been searched in a store, move forward.
27. If you were ever stopped or questioned by police about your presence in a particular neighborhood, take one step back.
28. Overall American women make 79% of the income of their male counterparts. Women, take one step back (2014 US Census Bureau).
29. As of 2015, black people made up only 4% of CEOs in Fortune 500 companies and women made only 4.8% (Berman 2015). All black people, and women take one step back.
30. If you have been called bad names because of your ethnicity, take one step back.
31. If you were raised in a home where a daily newspaper was delivered, take one step forward.
32. If you have ever been bullied in school for your race, gender, or sexual orientation, take one step back.
33. All who have been denied a job because of their race, ethnicity, or sexual orientation, take a step back.
34. If you had to hide your sexual orientation at any point in your life, for any reason, take a step back.
35. All those who ever inherited money or property, take one step forward.
36. All those who were told by their parents that they were beautiful, smart, and capable of achieving their dreams, take one step forward.
37. If you were ever physically, sexually, or emotionally abused as a child, take one step back.
38. If you ever had to escape your home country because of war, take one step back.
39. If you have ever been held in a refugee, concentration, or internment camp, take one step back.
40. All those who were raised in homes with children's and adult's books, take one step forward.

Questions Focused on Global Health

41. Twice the population of the United States (9% of the world's population) lives without access to safe water. Come to this side of the room if you have access to safe water.
42. Over 2.1 billion people in the developing world lived on less than US $ 3.10 a day in 2012 (29%). Take two steps forward if you make more than four dollars a day.
43. One in nine people does not have enough food to eat to lead a healthy life (www.wfp.org). Take one step forward if you have enough to eat to not go hungry (Energy Access Database).
44. In 2013, more than 2.7 billion people – 38% of the world's population – are estimated to have relied on the traditional use of solid biomass for cooking, typically using inefficient stoves in poorly ventilated spaces. Take one step

forward if you have a convenient gas stove in your kitchen (Energy Access Database). An estimated 1.2 billion people – 17% of the global population – did not have access to electricity in 2013, 84 million fewer than in the previous year.

References

Berman J (2015) Soon, not even 1 percent of fortune 500 Companies will have Black CEOs. http://www.huffingtonpost.com/2015/01/29/black-ceos-fortune-500_n_6572074.html Accessed 1 May 2018

Connor M (1994) Training the counsellor: an integrative model. Routledge, London

Energy Access Database. http://www.worldenergyoutlook.org/resources/energydevelopment/energyaccessdatabase/ Accessed 1 May 2018

Grant CA (ed) (1999) Multicultural research: race, class, gender and sexual orientation. Routledge Farmer, London

Halpern J (2003) What is Clinical Empathy? Journal of General Internal Medicine 18(8):670–674. https://doi.org/10.1046/j.1525-1497.2003.21017.x

Levinson WRD (1995) Physicians' psychosocial beliefs correlate with their patient communication skills. Journal of General Internal Medicine 10(7):375–379

Semuels A (2016) Poor at twenty, poor for life. The Atlantic. https://www.theatlantic.com/business/archive/2016/07/social-mobility-america/491240/ Accessed 1 May 2018

Shetty VU, Magliola R (2016) Sensitization as motivation: empowering first steps in global health. Paper presented at the AAFP Global Health Workshop. Atlanta, Georgia. https://resourcelibrary.stfm.org/viewdocument/sensitization-as-mot?CommunityKey=2751b51d-483f-45e2-81de-4faced0a290a&tab=librarydocuments

Shetty VU, Magliola R, Perzynski AT (2017) Proof of the pudding: impact of the horatio Alger exercise. Paper presented at the International Health Conference, Oxford, UK

Sue DW (2015) Race talk and facilitating difficult racial dialogues. Counseling Today, December 22, 2015. https://ct.counseling.org/2015/12/race-talk-and-facilitating-difficult-racial-dialogues/ Accessed 1 May 2018

Yeung M, Pliner E (2016) Race to the American Dream www.projectreachnyc.org/sites/all/themes/reach/.../RaceToTheAmericanDream.doc Accessed 1 May 2018

Teaching Social Determinants of Health

Megan Rich

Social Determinants of Health Curriculum Description: A Longitudinal Structure

The following curriculum was created specifically for the training of family medicine and family medicine-psychiatry combined residents at University of Cincinnati/ Christ Hospital in Cincinnati, OH. The faculty champion for the social determinants of health (SDH) training program began curriculum redesign by performing a needs assessment, including exploring the literature for published best practices, reviewing Accreditation Council of Graduate Medical Education (ACGME) common program requirements for residencies including the family medicine milestones project, and interviewing leadership within the residency and clinic for insight into their vision of trainee competency caring for vulnerable populations. The resulting construct was an amalgam of pertinent knowledge, skills, and attitudes needed to train our residents with special emphasis on the SDH. Although this structure was optimized for medical trainees, there are certain elements that are relevant and useful as is or via adaptation for other health professionals.

The subsequent SDH program outcomes, written based on the needs assessment results, can be categorized in two key behaviors: identifying the SDH and addressing the SDH, as shown in Box 1. Both behaviors can be performed on behalf of or in partnership with individual patients and entire communities. Primary and secondary objectives needed to accomplish the outcomes were identified and teaching methods were developed to meet the objectives.

The program was designed to take place over the course of 3 years. It was intentionally developed to introduce different components at key times of development.

M. Rich (✉)
Department of Family & Community Medicine, University of Cincinnati,
Cincinnati, OH, USA
e-mail: richma@ucmail.uc.edu

© The Author(s) 2019
A. Perzynski et al. (eds.), *Health Disparities*,
https://doi.org/10.1007/978-3-030-12771-8_59

Box 1: SDH Longitudinal Curriculum Outcomes

To identify SDH, residents should be able to		To address SDH, residents should be able to	
Primary Objectives	Secondary Objectives	Primary Objectives	Secondary Objectives
Recall descriptions of the SDH and their impact they have on health	Identify the social, environmental, and cultural barriers to health in individual patients across multiple clinical sites.	Identify community resources to address SDH	List community resources that can assist in addressing the four most common SDH within the FMC
	Explain the impact on health of each of the following: access to care culture race violence and adverse childhood events education and health literacy occupation income housing food insecurity/nutrition incarceration undocumented status	Collaborate with patients and families in generating a plan to address SDH	Incorporate biological and social factors and appropriate community resources into a treatment plan
Ask about the presence of SDH in a way that elicits an honest response from the patient	Take a sensitive and patient-centered social history including screening for the SDH	Recognize the role of advocacy in creating solutions for SDH at a community level	Describe an example of a physician who has advocated for a specific SDH
	Practice specific communication techniques to bridge cultural and experiential differences		
Integrate SDH screening questions into the office visit	Document identified SDH in the electronic medical record	Modify current office processes in a way that enhances the ability of doctors and staff to address SDH	Evaluate current office processes that impact SDH and implement a change
	Perform pre-visit planning with the medical assistant, specifically identifying patients that will need screening for presence of SDH		

Interns, for instance, have curriculum components that focus on ensuring a sound foundation of knowledge about health disparities of the communities they serve and local resources. They are exposed to patient perspectives of the SDH and health equity as they continue to develop their attitudes about what it means to be a physician caring for the underserved. Basic communication skills including practicing culturally sensitive interviewing techniques are also introduced.

As residents progress in their training and earn more autonomy, the focus shifts from predominantly teaching knowledge to developing and refining skill sets. Deliberate practice—the cycle of practice with feedback followed by practice again in rapid succession—is key here, as is ensuring that residents see the link between what they are learning and patient care. Thus, the objectives shift to incorporating SDH into their patient care activities. Preceptors are prompted to provide this feedback through an online form that includes a question about observed resident behaviors in identifying and addressing SDH during the office session. This is also a time to refine communication skills. Social needs can be a sensitive topic of discussion, and the use of specific communication strategies to ease these conversations is an objective of the curriculum.

Thus far, the emphasis of SDH teaching has mostly been on the individual patient and doctor-patient dyad. During their third and final year of training, the SDH program shifts to encourage residents to consider how to identify and address SDH at a population level. One valuable teaching method is the incorporation of quality improvement projects and methodology to explore office processes that hinder or help in the diagnosing and treating of health-related social needs. Currently, this is an opt-in project with roughly a quarter of the residents involved, all of them in the final 2 years of their training. The final step in actualizing physicians with robust training in SDH is incorporating advocacy and community engagement. While it is certainly relevant to the work of primary care doctors to know how to connect individuals to community resources, engaging in activism to promote public health at a local, state, or national level is important for the health of the communities in which we serve.

Design of Educational Strategies

Teaching strategies to enhance intern knowledge of health disparities include a health disparities workshop during intern orientation. This consists of introducing to state, county, and neighborhood data on current disparities and comparisons to neighboring states and counties. SDH-related data from the resident continuity office is shared. The structure of the session is interactive: working in pairs, interns spend time at multiple stations with question prompts that elicit examination of printouts or websites with relevant information. Interns return for a group debriefing and the focus shifts to a big picture discussion of why health inequities exist and consideration of the physician's role and professional responsibilities to improve health equity.

Every October, interns are pulled from traditional clinical rotations to participate in a "boot camp" of sorts, including (but not limited to) activities teaching on SDH. During this time, the interns are scheduled for a group outing into a neighborhood surrounding the clinic. The SDH Field Experience is a community experience where residents visit social service agencies such as a food bank, charitable pharmacy, and the county welfare and Medicaid office, hearing first hand from workers and clients. It is an opportunity not only to get to know the city and one of the neighborhoods their patients commonly live in, but to explore how, when, and why to connect a patient to the community resource. The experience includes a requirement to take public transportation and culminates with reflection through the exploration of learner-generated photographs and written reflection.

Also incorporated into the October Intern Boot Camp is a didactic session on culturally competent interviewing. We teach the BATHE technique for its universality and ability to navigate differences in life experiences, even between two people from the same country or culture (Lieberman and Stuart 1999). It is also a quick method that can easily be incorporated into an office visit. The teaching session uses role-play and active participation with peer feedback to help learners get comfortable with the technique.

For residents in their second year of training, teaching is through intentional modeling and feedback from preceptors who observe the residents caring for their panel of continuity patients. Preceptors specifically look for indications that the resident incorporated any identified SDH into the care plan. Feedback is sent to the residents electronically.

During their final year in training, senior residents are invited to participate in an examination of office processes related to the SDH. Currently, there are no standard procedures for screening, identifying, or responding to known SDH that are negatively impacting the health of patients. This is a quality improvement initiative, as there is much data to suggest that the SDH have a bigger impact on health outcomes than writing a prescription (Crawford 2018).

Some activities are designed for the participation of all available residents (regardless of training level) because they address many of the primary objectives at once or because of limited resources to target a specific level of training. For instance, all available trainees attend an annual lecture on advocacy. This lecture can target many different aspects of advocacy and the resident group in attendance can choose the advocacy topic. For the past 2 years, the residents have chosen to focus on activism including talking to politicians and exploring state and local legislative bills that impact health.

Every 18 months available residents participate in a 1.5-hour workshop called The Community Resource Fair. Representatives from six local social service agencies are invited to attend. Residents are divided into four teams of six and each given a separate patient scenario. One person from each group visits one of the six agencies, interviewing the agency representative and then reports back to their original team about the ways in which an agency could or could not help the patient in their scenario. It culminates with each team creating a comprehensive care plan, presenting the plan to the large group, and hearing from the agency representatives about any misconceptions or clarifications.

Evaluating the Curriculum

The evaluation plan includes examining resident attitudes and behaviors. The ideal outcome is a physician with knowledge, skills, and attitudes to practice medicine in a socially informed way. During our multifaceted evaluation, we examine knowledge through a pre- and posttest, attitudes through an annual survey and written reflections, and behavior through observation of clinical activities and a chart review of social needs documentation practices within the health record.

During an office session, the residents receive feedback from the precepting faculty member via an electronic evaluation form. One question on the form asks specifically about the level of independence the resident demonstrated around the SDH: "Resident identifies a social determinant of health (such as housing safety, food insecurity, violence, racism/discrimination) when causing major impact on patient's health status and adjusts treatment plan accordingly." This is linked to several Family Medicine Milestones (systems based practice, professionalism, and interpersonal communication) (ACGME and ABFM 2015).

An additional method of programmatic evaluation includes performing chart reviews of resident office visit notes and problem lists in the medical record. In many clinical settings there is no standardized procedure for documenting social needs in the medical records of our patients. There are now ICD-10 codes relating to social needs Torres, et al. ICD Social Codes: An Underutilized Resource for Tracking Social Needs (2017), a potential new way to document and track SDH. The results of a pilot study in which we reviewed a random sampling of resident and faculty charts showed most physicians in our office are documenting social needs in the social history. None in the sample incorporated socials needs into the problem list, nor utilized ICD-10 codes. It is unlikely this small study will capture all resident behaviors but it can give a sample of conversation topics and their frequency.

Future Directions

Not all precepting faculty practice at the residency continuity clinic. Thus, one of the next phases of the curriculum will incorporate faculty development for preceptors. This is especially important as modeling, such as when precepting, is an important teaching tool particularly for care of underserved patients.

Conversations around social needs are crucial ones, requiring some finesse to take the perspective of the patient and foster a relationship based on trust and mutual respect. The best teaching method is one of observation, feedback, and reflection. Using video or audio recordings, residents can listen to their conversations, self-critique, share with faculty for additional feedback, and then implement changes. Patient consent is needed to record the encounter and resident enthusiasm for this method of teaching has been low in the past. Faculty time to listen and assess conversations is another barrier that needs to be considered.

Example Teaching Method #1: SDH and Health Disparities Workshop (Fig. 1)

The health disparities workshop, given annually during intern orientation, serves as an introduction for new trainees. In addition to examining health disparities and key public health issues at the state, county, city/neighborhood level, interns also become familiar with the layout of the city and surrounding communities. At times, we share important history such as the closing of a grocery store which created a food desert. The goal is for interns to connect the dots between health disparities and current public health initiatives as well as the social determinants of health.

Health disparities are sometimes presented as a laundry list of statistics, yet this hardly seems the best method for transformative learning. The teaching method used here tries to avoid disengaged learners by structuring the learning session to have active manipulation of the data in teams of two. By working with a partner, we hope to promote discussion and deeper learning.

Step 1: Plan the Session

For a successful health disparities workshop, faculty investment in preparation is critical. The faculty lead for the session compiles data from various sources. For instance, reports from the Ohio Department Health, Hamilton County Public Health, and the Cincinnati Health Department are gathered from their websites. Community

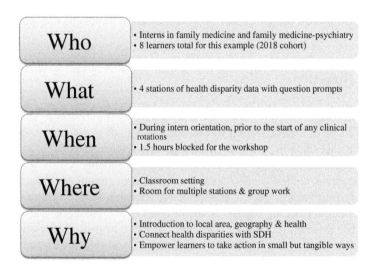

Fig. 1 The Five W's of a health disparities and social determinants of health (SDH) workshop

needs assessments are included when available. For the past two years, we have included population data based on zip codes of patients in the residency clinic as well as patient responses to questionnaires and interviews about screening for the social needs. In the latest iteration, three of the four stations included an interactive website.

The amount of data from an array of resources can be overwhelming, so choices must be made about which topics to pursue. Once data and topics are selected, the faculty lead creates question prompts (about 3–5) for each station. This guides the learners attention as they examine the data and statistics, and prompts self-reflection about how their own office and personal behaviors as a physician might evolve.

Objectives for SDOH and Health Disparities Workshop

- Familiarize yourselves with the Cincinnati community including examination of local geography, health disparities, and public health issues.
- Describe the connection between health disparities and the social determinants of health (SDH).
- Compare key population characteristics (gender, race, insurance type) to local health disparities.
- Consider future interventions you might take to ensure health equity for all (Figs. 2 and 3).

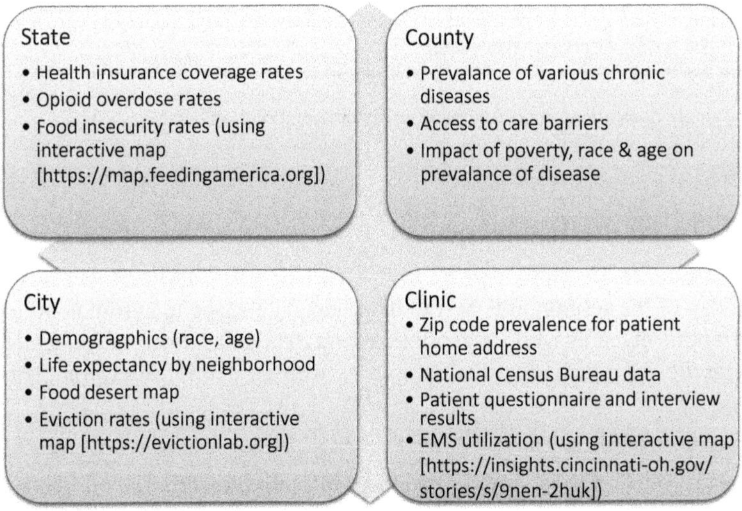

State
- Health insurance coverage rates
- Opioid overdose rates
- Food insecurity rates (using interactive map [https://map.feedingamerica.org])

County
- Prevalance of various chronic diseases
- Access to care barriers
- Impact of poverty, race & age on prevalance of disease

City
- Demogragphics (race, age)
- Life expectancy by neighborhood
- Food desert map
- Eviction rates (using interactive map [https://evictionlab.org])

Clinic
- Zip code prevalence for patient home address
- National Census Bureau data
- Patient questionnaire and interview results
- EMS utilization (using interactive map [https://insights.cincinnati-oh.gov/stories/s/9nen-2huk])

Fig. 2 Levels of data sources for social determinants and health disparities

---

County Data: Sample Question Prompts

1. Begin with the Community Health Status Survey [https://www.interactforhealth.org/upl/media/chss17_methodology_final_050917.pdf] results. Do you see any links between perceived health of the region and having a primary care doctor (or office)?
    - Now look at the obesity rates, child behaviors, and county-level data of chronic disease prevalence (depicted in maps). In what ways do these data confirm or dispute the overall perceived health of Hamilton County?
2. Insurance coverage rates in Ohio have improved in the past couple years. But having insurance does not mean that there are no longer barriers to accessing healthcare services. Take a look at the graphs depicting responses from patients ("consumer stakeholders") as well as agencies (i.e. nonprofit organizations servicing underserved, low income and minority populations) and the health department. What are the barriers from the patient's perspective? From the community agency and health department perspectives? Are there any barriers that are specific for Latinos?
3. How do income and educational attainment impact PERCEIVED health?
4. Do you think that a patient's income, race or educational attainment are things a doctor should know or ask about?

City/Neighborhood Data: Sample Question Prompts

1. Let's begin by examining demographic data of the city. How dose the city's profile compare to Hamilton County for age and race?
2. Examine the life expectancy map and chart. Find the FMC's neighborhood (Mt Auburn). What is the difference in life expectancy (as measured in years) between the following communities:
    - Mt Auburn & Over-The-Rhine
    - Clifton & Avondale
    - Mt Lookout & Linwood
    - Your neighborhood (if you live within city limits) and Mt Auburn
3. Food deserts (as defined by the USDA) are "parts of the country vapid of fresh fruit, vegetables, and other healthful whole foods, usually found in impoverished areas. This is largely due to a lack of grocery stores, farmers' markets, and healthy food providers." Using the map, find your own neighborhood. Is there a grocery store (blue dot) near you? How do you get to the grocery store?
    - Walnut Hills doesn't have a grocery store anymore (see news story in references). Mt Lookout doesn't have a grocery store in the neighborhood either. How is the burden of accessing food different for these two communities?

Fig. 3 Sample question prompts for county, city, and neighborhood data

Step 2: Teach the Workshop

On the day of the session, it is best to have adequate space to ensure nondisruptive conversations in teams while at the stations and a room large enough to comfortably lead a group introduction to the activity as well as debrief after completing the stations.

A suggested format for the session is as follows:

- Minutes 0–10: Large group introduction using PowerPoint or white board. Communicate purpose/objectives, define key vocabulary (health disparity vs health equity, equity vs equality), and explain how the activity will work. Administer pretest if giving one.

- Minutes 10–25: Time at station 1. Divide learners into pairs and have each pair start at a different station. Provide handout with question prompts to each individual. Make sure data materials are printed out and available at each station. If using online interactive maps, ensure tablet or computer is available at each station and pulled up to correct website.
- Minutes 25–40: Time at station 2. Have learners rotate to the next station. If they haven't finished all the questions, have them move on anyway.
- Minutes 40–55: Time at station 3.
- Minutes 55–70: Time at station 4.
- Minutes 70–90: Return to large group for debrief. Lead facilitated discussion to get learners discussing data they found surprising, intriguing, and/or upsetting. Ask learners to identify strengths of communities traditionally thought of as "disadvantaged." Lead learners to discuss practical steps that they can take to address disparities they noted (e.g., screening for food insecurity at well child checks, adding tobacco use to problem list and checking in with patient at each visit, keeping syphilis on the differential diagnosis). As time allows, have learners commit to one thing by writing it down on a notecard. Administer posttest if using.

Materials Needed for Day of Workshop

- Printouts of question prompts, enough for each learner
- Data and statistic resources printed out and categorized for each station
- Computer or tablet at stations utilizing interactive maps, screen open to website
- PowerPoint slides (if using)
- Pre- and posttest questions (if using)
- Timer
- Notecards
- Evaluation form of the session to be completed by learners (can be incorporated to posttest)

Step 3: Evaluate the Workshop

As the primary objective for this learning session is to enhance knowledge (more so than skills or attitudes), a written assessment was deemed the best assessment method. The 2018 intern cohort was given an online 10-question pre- and posttest. Questions were both short answer and multiple choice, and the faculty lead for the session graded the tests. The posttest included an extra four questions for learner reaction to the session, eliciting feedback for possible future improvements.

Example Teaching Method #2: Social Determinants of Health Field Experience (Fig. 4)

The social determinants of health (SDH) field experience has been taught annually for more than a decade, taking interns (along with one or two faculty members) into the neighborhoods where many of the resident patients live and meeting with social workers, clients, and executive directors of government and nonprofit organizations that provide services to the poor. The objectives for this activity include enhancing knowledge of community resources and appropriate channels to access offered service, evolving attitudes about what it means to care for marginalized populations, and the act of experiencing some of the barriers to accessing health care that resident patients may have to navigate. Objectives should be individualized to each program and based on an understanding of which SDH are most common for the patients served by the trainees. This can be determined by examining zip codes and National Census Bureau data or through discussions with representatives from the partner service organizations and/or patients from the clinic.

Objectives for SDH Field Experience

- Identify and navigate commonly used community resources as they relate to our continuity clinic patient population.
- Appreciate (be aware of) the patient perspective when accessing health care.
- Experience transportation as a determinant of health.

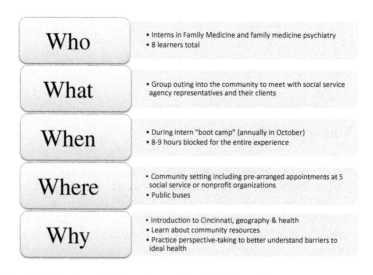

Fig. 4 The Five W's of a social determinants of health field experience

Field Experience Implementation

Similar field experiences have been previously described in the literature with various spins on activities and teaching methods incorporated into the outing. For instance, some variations include a budgeting activity [Klein, et al. Training in Social Determinants of Health in Primary Care: Does it Change Resident Behavior? Academic pediatrics, 2011], incorporate a poverty simulation [Wallace, et al. An Experiential Community Orientation to Improve Knowledge and Assess Resident Attitudes Toward Poor Patients JGME 2013], feature culturally or historically important locations [Patow, et al Who's in Our Neighborhood? Healthcare Disparities Experiential Education for Residents Ochsner Journal 2016] or focus on the voices of community leaders and activists [Fornari, et al Learning Social Medicine in the Bronx: An Orientation for Primary Care Residents Teaching & learning in Medicine 2011; Chang, et al The Impact of "See the City You Serve" Field Trip: An Educational Tool for Teaching Social Determinants of Health JGME 2017]. Our variation includes two special components: the requirement that public transportation be used to get to appointments and the assignment of taking photographs of environments or behaviors that affirm or detract from the health of communities.

While other programs have described using buses to transport learners during field experiences [Fornari, et al Learning Social Medicine in the Bronx: An Orientation for Primary Care Residents Teaching & learning in Medicine 2011; Chang, et al The Impact of "See the City You Serve" Field Trip: An Educational Tool for Teaching Social Determinants of Health JGME 2017], the buses described are charter buses servicing only those on the learning activity. In our experience, we utilize the public busing system, exposing residents to the benefits and challenges of that mode of transportation. Using public transportation our residents have experienced the tardiness of buses and the complexity of the bus system including the need to transfer to another bus line. For some of our learners, it is their first experience using public transportation. Interns are provided with a gift card to cover expenses including bus fare and lunch, although they are advised that they cannot use the gift card to buy a bus ticket so they should bring cash or download the app and pay electronically (using the app also has teachable moments as it does not always work as well as one would hope) (Fig. 5).

The second unique component of the experience is that residents are asked to use photography to capture compelling moments throughout the morning. They are prompted at the outset to seek out examples of health promoting or hindering behaviors, environments or conditions, and/or services. Guidelines are reviewed including the need to get permission from any person included in a photograph and safety suggestions. The purpose of the photographs is not to judge any single person or community, but to gather insight to the learner and why they chose to capture the scene within the photograph. The learners present their photographs and talk about the meaning behind them as a part of the group debriefing in the afternoon. This discussion is recorded on video.

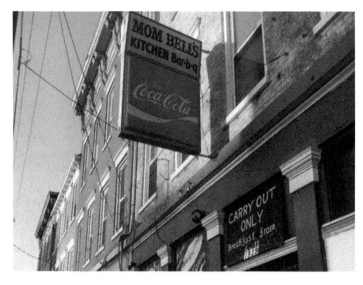

Fig. 5 Example of food options in a local Cincinnati neighborhood

Field Experience Evaluation

We evaluate the experience both through learner reaction and a thematic analysis of resident generated documents. Learner reaction is collected through anonymous but mandatory electronic questionnaire which include five questions about specific sites visited, logistics, and teaching impact. This evaluation by learners specific to the SDH field experience has only been in place for 1 year resulting in a very small sample size. Prior to creation of this form, learners were able to give feedback as a part of the more generic rotation evaluation form (also online, anonymous and compulsory).

The attitudinal development of our learners is at the heart of the SDH field experience. To try and capture the evolving attitudes of the interns, we have begun analysis of the resident reflections and intend to do a qualitative study on the transcripts of the photo debrief videos as well as on the photographs themselves. Initial results of the thematic analysis of the reflections are shared below. Sample size remains relatively small ($N = 15$) and thus data collection and analysis are ongoing.

As with all qualitative research, the lens through which the researchers view the data is important to note. The author uses a critical action research social justice framework which includes the belief that research should be a call to action [Merriam & Tisdell Qualitative research: a guide to design and implementation, 4th Ed. Jossey-Bass 2016]. As an educator she also incorporates a constructivist perspective, the belief that learning is constructed through experience and interaction with others [Merriam, et al Learning in Adulthood: a comprehensive guide, 3rd Ed. Jossey-Bass 2007]. The process of reviewing included anonymizing each reflection and then two researchers independently reviewing all 15 reflections, generating themes, and identifying quotes to represent each them. Disputes were settled by the lead researcher who also identified overarching global themes.

Three primary themes were identified: content learned, learning processes, and learner reactions. The content learned theme included descriptions of social services and social determinants of health. The learning process themes encompassed stories of patients (as interns connected the day's events with past learning), future application (comments on how they might change their practice), evolving attitudes (including stereotype of poverty), and taking another's perspective (imaging how their patients might feel). The final theme, learner reaction, included a variety of responses to the experience including emotional reactions and feedback for the teachers. Similar types of themes have been noted by others [Wallace, et al An Experiential Community Orientation to Improve Knowledge and Assess Resident Attitudes Toward Poor Patients JGME 2013; Chang, et al The Impact of "See the City You Serve" Field Trip: An Educational Tool for Teaching Social Determinants of Health JGME 2017] (Fig. 6).

While we intend to continue with this teaching method, additional changes may be incorporated in the future. This includes intentional teaching around historically and culturally relevant landmarks and to call out the strengths and assets of the neighborhoods we visit. An outing such as this one always runs the risk of becoming "medical tourism" where we, the visitors, peer into communities as if they are an exhibit. Gregg and coauthors [health and disease in context] argue that longitudinal curricula continue to push residents out of their comfort zones throughout training which is one way to avoid the medical tourism trap. Faculty during the outing can

Example Content Learned Quote
"One fact that stood out in my mind is that although there are resources available, it is a long process to securing them; I wish there were more emergency safety nets in place for families who cannot wait."

Reflection 11

Example Learner Reaction Quote
"The emotions I experienced on our day...are a mix of joy for the resilience and hope that people (especially young people) are capable of, as well as sadness and frustration over the unjust structures of our economic systems that lock some into cycles of poverty while allowing others to amass more and more wealth."

Reflection 5

Example Learning Processes Quote
"I won't naively say that one day out in the community in the rain makes me appreciate all the strife and frustration that my patients experience each and every day, but it did remind me that it's important to change perspectives, empathize with others and keep on working to connect with the community to understand everyone a bit better."

Reflection 15

Fig. 6 Example quotes from field experience learners

also mitigate this by using teachable moments to reinforce the assets of low-resource communities and to stress the importance of collaboration with the community in finding ways to raise the level of health for all.

Example Teaching Method #3: Incorporating Social Determinants of Health into Office Quality Improvement Activities (Fig. 7)

Background

Research by Bazemore and colleagues describes a process that each practice can undertake to better understand our patients and the populations we serve and then to develop action steps to better serve them (Bazemore et al. 2015). The first step is to know your patient population. They suggest starting with zip code data. This is where we began. Utilizing our technology resources of the electronic medical record, we pulled all the zip codes of the 7000-plus patients established in the Family Medicine Center (FMC). This spreadsheet of numbers (no other patient data was pulled) was then uploaded into an online geo-spatial mapping tool called

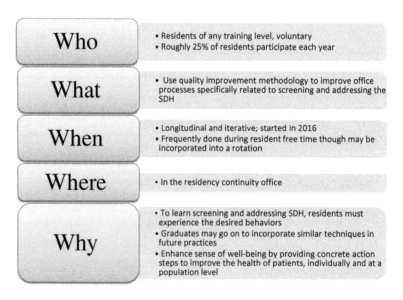

Fig. 7 The Five W's of incorporating social determinants into office-based quality improvement

HealthLandscape [https://www.healthlandscape.org/About.cfm]. This tool created a map of patient home address by zip code, identifying the zip codes where patient homes were most concentrated.

Once we had the most common zip codes, we could then utilize other resources such as the Vulnerable Populations Footprint Tool (https://assessment.community-commons.org/Footprint/l). This public and free data gave us insight to the possible barriers for people living in each zip code including transportation (such as lack of vehicle ownership), high school graduation rates, and average income. Not every social need is evaluated., but there are increasing tools to investigate neighborhoods using geocoding. Evictionlab.org is one example: its interactive web-based map gives eviction rate information by census tract. Users comfortable with the R-programming language can utilize a new tool called "Sociome" (https://github.com/NikKrieger/sociome) which allows users to generate data and a map of the Area Deprivation index for any community in the United States using any year of the American Community Survey from the U.S. Census.

The other way to garner insight into the social needs of a patient panel is to ask the patients. We created a survey using screening questions from various validated SDH questionnaires as well as some demographic data. We administered the survey to adult patients who were waiting for their appointment. The results helped us to understand which social needs are most prevalent according to our patients' reported experiences. The questionnaires were followed up by semi-structured interviews done in person or via phone.

Future Action

As we continue to move forward in finding a way to implement SDH screening processes in a way that is respectful and patient centered, we plan to rely on input from our patient and family advisory council, especially when considering the logistics. For example, should the questions be asked in person, on paper, or online? During an office visit? Before arriving for the visit? Clinic staff specifically have voiced enthusiasm for the project and including them in discussions of the best methods for streamlining and standardizing such screening will be important. Algorithms for follow-up questions and responses to positive screens would need to be completed before screening can be implemented. We plan to begin with a pilot, screening a specific patient population within the office rather than launching comprehensive screening of all patients. This might be patients with a high burden of chronic disease (such as patients with a hemoglobin A1c over 9) or added to an already standardized visit (such as at the 12-month well-child visit). Once the process for screening a small patient sample has been established, we can begin to consider implementation for the large office population.

References

Accreditation Council for Graduate Medical Education and The American Board of Family Medicine 2015 The Family Medicine Milestone Project https://www.acgme.org/Portals/0/PDFs/Milestones/FamilyMedicineMilestones.pdf Accessed September 1, 2018

Bazemore AW, Cottrell EK, Gold R, Hughes LS, Phillips RL, Angier H, Burdick TE, Carrozza MA, DeVoe JE (2015) "Community vital signs": incorporating geocoded social determinants into electronic records to promote patient and population health. Journal of the American Medical Informatics Association;23(2):407-412

Crawford C (2018) The EveryONE Project Unveils Social Determinants of Health Tools. American Association of Family Physicians https://www.aafp.org/news/health-of-the-public/20180109sdohtools.html. Accessed 31 Aug 2018

Lieberman III JA, Stuart MR (1999) The BATHE method: Incorporating counseling and psychotherapy into the everyday management of patients. Primary care companion to the Journal of clinical psychiatry;1(2):35

The Wheels of Misfortune

Adam Perzynski

This activity is based off of the general concept and method of the Wheel of Fortune™ game. You will need a chalkboard, whiteboard, or touch screen. Draw a large circle, and leave sufficient space to write words as "wedges" or sections in the circle. The exercise is simple and can be used for small or large groups of learners. There are three basic steps (Fig. 1).

1. Gather the group of students/participants and have them pair up with one other person. Ask them to identify what social, behavioral, or cultural factors could be seen as causes or drivers of health disparities? Give them 1 minute to complete this task.
2. Have each group give their answers. Write the answers in sequence onto the first wheel. Take this opportunity to clarify the meaning of terms and share information about how each category affects health (e.g., socioeconomic status, gender, etc.).
3. Repeat the first two steps; only this time, have the pairs identify health conditions diseases or care processes wherein disparities might be experienced (e.g., infant mortality, blood pressure control). Use the second wheel for writing the answers. This step can be used as an opportunity to promote critical questions and will often result in participants questioning whether there really is a disparity present for the conditions that their peers mention.
4. Ask participants their reaction overall to viewing so many social factors and so many conditions on the two respective wheels. An important point for the facilitator to make during the discussion is that as a person moves through life; they get multiple "spins" on both wheels. The exercise can be a powerful illustration of how the accumulation of health and social disadvantage is not linear and that social and health problems can beget additional health and social problems.

A. Perzynski (✉)
Center for Health Care Research and Policy, The MetroHealth System,
Case Western Reserve University, Cleveland, OH, USA
e-mail: Adam.Perzynski@case.edu

© The Author(s) 2019   237
A. Perzynski et al. (eds.), *Health Disparities*,
https://doi.org/10.1007/978-3-030-12771-8_60

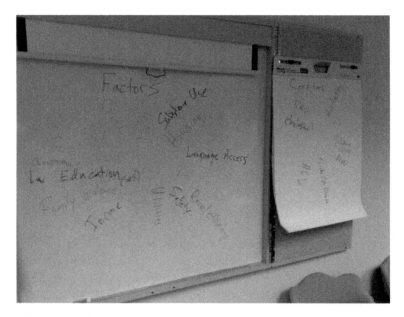

Fig. 1 Wheels of misfortune from a seminar with primary care faculty

Brief Guide to Writing Case Narratives

Sarah Shick, Ifeolorunbode Adebambo, and Adam Perzynski

Why Create Case Narratives of Health Disparities?

Narratives are awesome! They emphasize a depth of understanding and tie abstract ideas to real life. Narratives have long been a tradition in both medicine and social science. At the 2018 meeting of the Society for Longitudinal and Life Course Studies in Milan, Italy, sociologist Dr. Ross MacMillan asked the gathered scientists, "What kind of data can establish causality?" After much debate, the only consensus was that a rich qualitative narrative was best suited to determining the presence causality in human interactions. Case narratives help us to develop the concepts and relationships between concepts that form the foundation for theory and change. This section will provide you with some tools to write your own case narratives.

Different Types of Case Narratives

- *Extreme Cases*: Extraordinary or unusual person or situation. The study of outliers can better help us to understand normalcy (Fritz 2008).

S. Shick
Department of Sociology, Case Western Reserve University, Center for Health Care Research and Policy, The MetroHealth System, Cleveland, OH, USA

I. Adebambo
Department of Family Medicine, The MetroHealth System, Cleveland, OH, USA

A. Perzynski (✉)
Center for Health Care Research and Policy, The MetroHealth System, Case Western Reserve University, Cleveland, OH, USA
e-mail: Adam.Perzynski@case.edu

© The Author(s) 2019
A. Perzynski et al. (eds.), *Health Disparities*,
https://doi.org/10.1007/978-3-030-12771-8_61

- *Paradigmatic Cases*: Exemplifies specific concepts and principles. Often based in patterns of behavior or circumstances (Fritz 2008).
- *Critical Cases:* These cases are most often used to test or develop theories. They are typically selected carefully to illustrate a particular circumstance, experience, or event and build a common understanding (Fritz 2008).

Considerations for Writing Cases

Balancing creative writing and the demands of undergraduate, graduate, postgraduate, or continuing education can be difficult. Don't worry about it—if you're participating in this program, you have definitely survived worse! Here are some tips to help you write a case narrative.

Writer Anne Lamott has suggested in her book of the same title that writers go "bird by bird," one piece of the story at a time (Lamott 2007). You will most likely write what Anne called "shitty first drafts," and that is not only acceptable, but encouraged. Accept that perfection is impossible, especially on the first try.

Most often one of the important components of good writing, and of powerful case narratives, is to give the reader the context of the story that is unfolding. The adage in the writing world is "show don't tell," and it allows the reader to use their imagination to visualize what you are describing, thus making your writing more engaging. We advise our clinician writers against solely using analytical language as they would in clinical notes. Instead we ask them to offer deeper details that can reflect on the character of the patient and the context of the clinic.

Yes, this is an African American woman in her mid-40s with rheumatoid arthritis, schizophrenia, and complex gynecological history. But does she have silver-white hair—is it in long braids or a stylish bob? Are her eyes kind and soft, shifting nervously, or perhaps distant and forlorn? Does she have a belly laugh that gives you a smile, or is she timid and hard to understand through a thick southern accent? Is this a clinic in the hospital with all of the newest equipment or is it an inner-city satellite clinic in a long line of storefront shops facing a battered parking lot full of potholes? These kinds of valuable details are often part of the memory of an encounter and can convey a far clearer and more engaging retelling of the situation.

Writing a strong description of who, when, and where can be fun—use your imagination if you can't remember a small detail like if her shirt was orange or yellow, but stay as true to life as much as possible. Feel free to use your favorite word from the dictionary, but keep your use of language accessible and relatively simple. Thick, enticing descriptions will show the power of your writing far better than long strings of 5–7 syllable words.

Avoid "blowbyblow" of events writing. Few people enjoy reading, "Then repairman left. Then Judge Judy came on, you know how I like her. Then I put on my arthritis cream. Oh, and then the kitty needed its tuna and milk, so I got out of my chair and…" You get the point. Don't drone on, for all of our sakes! Giving context and rich descriptions to the patient, the interaction, and the location will make it more fun for everyone.

Helpful Questions for Writers of Case Narratives

- What is the background of the person and the situation?
- What is their family and social situation?
- Are there important organizational conditions or social determinants of health?

  - Insurance
  - Transportation issues
  - Worker's compensation injured worker status
  - Underfunded, inadequate, or difficult to access services needed by patient?

- How are other clinic staff members interacting with the patient? Is it different than your interaction?
- What is unique to this case?
- What is similar to other cases?
- What assertions or generalizations can we make?
- Was there something that stuck with you or changed the way you practice?

You're Ready to Start Now!

Write a draft knowing you can go back and make it better. Start by writing down what you want to say. You will need to begin to make some decisions (albeit reversible ones of little consequence for now):

- Type of disparities to write about:

  - Gender
  - Race/ethnicity
  - Class or socioeconomic position
  - Age
  - Disability
  - Language barrier
  - Technology
  - Education
  - Insurance/social services
  - Many or all of the above?
  - Others?

- *Type of case*

  - Extreme
  - Paradigmatic
  - Critical

If you feel stuck, consider that taking a walk has been shown to help creativity, and writing with a pen and paper instead of your computer can jar your brain and your thinking and can possibly help by changing the flow of words and prompting you to write differently. Share a story of a patient or circumstance that really hit you and can influence clinical practice—one from years ago or one from yesterday. There is no "right" answer. Consider that the majority of what you read on a regular basis has a bunch of highly educated and experienced editors helping the piece reach publishable perfection, so don't bother to hold yourself to that standard, just let it be inspiration. Use this guide, and the references listed below, to help you as you tell your story of interacting with a patient facing a health disparity. Best wishes, and happy writing!

Reference

Lamott A (2007) Bird by bird: some instructions on writing and life. Anchor, Norwell
Fritz K (2008) Case study and narrative analysis. The Johns Hopkins University. Available: http://ocw.jhsph.edu/courses/QualitativeDataAnalysis/PDFs/Session4.pdf

Index

CPSIA information can be obtained
at www.ICGtesting.com
Printed in the USA
LVHW080927070222
710433LV00001B/4

9 783030 127732